Herbal Antibiotics

Learn the Secrets of Natural Remedies Using Medicinal Herbs (2022 Guide for Beginners)

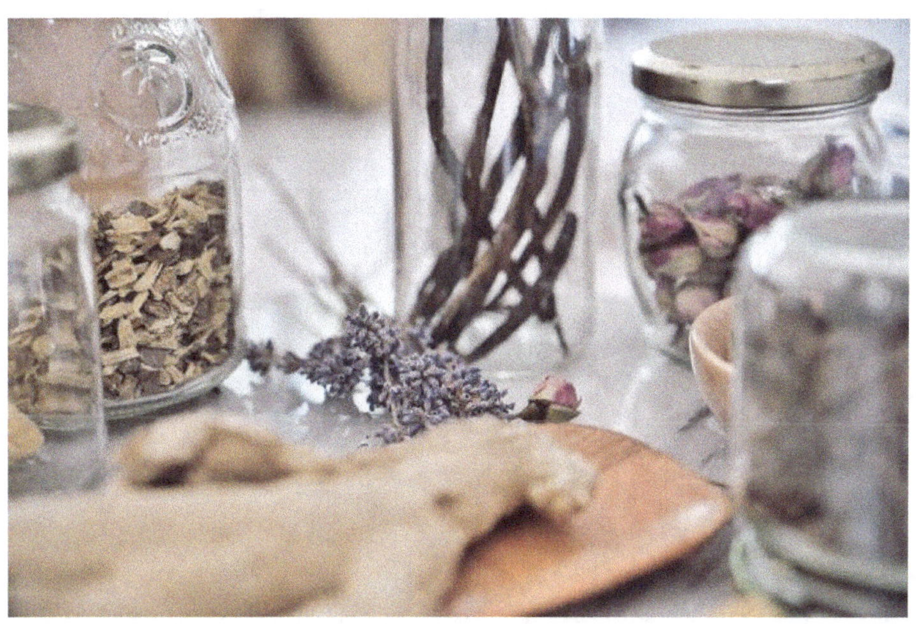

Bud Abbott

Table of Contents

Herbal antibiotics aid in the development of immunological reserves and immunodeficiency, which improves health and quality of life. Herbal concoctions have the potential to be effective against drug-resistant microorganisms. It has a high level of immunological activation because it activates white blood cells to fight bacterial and viral illnesses. It also stimulates the synthesis of interferon, a protein that protects cells from viral invasion.

Bacteria, viruses, poisons, parasites, and microorganisms are all protected by the immune system. It is critical to maintaining a healthy immune system. Infections, colds and flu, cancer, and heart disease are all more likely among people who have a weakened immune system. Bacteria can be found everywhere, and hundreds of good germs dwell in the human body, helping to defend it against harmful bacteria. Antibiotics are effective against bad bacteria, but they also kill healthy bacteria. Good bacteria, which line the digestive, respiratory, and urinary tracts, play a crucial role in the immune system. The use of prescription antibiotics frequently results in increased yeast development, which weakens the immune system even further.

Herbs can help purify and detoxify the body while also supporting excellent blood chemistry. The body receives what it requires to withstand, repair, and overcome ailments and reach Optimal Health by nourishing and harmonizing the system. Antibiotic herbs are effective against bacteria, viruses, and fungi. Treatment may not be as quick as medicine. Although antibiotic herbs are gentler than medicines, they should only be used when absolutely required. Antibiotics on prescription will always be available when we need them.

Some Fundamentals of Natural Antibiotics

We believe that everyone should have a basic understanding of natural antibiotics. This would entail understanding natural chemicals having antibiotic capabilities as well as how to use them to generate the antibiotic effect.

Before getting into our arguments for why we believe everyone should have a basic understanding of natural antibiotics, we must first provide a brief overview of the concept of antibiotics in general and natural antibiotics in particular.

Antibiotics are now compounds used to combat germs. Bacteria, as we all know, are microorganisms (mostly fungus and viruses) that cause disease. Bacteria are probably responsible for more diseases than any other sort of microorganism. Of course, not all microorganisms cause disease. There are bacteria that are really beneficial to us, microorganisms whose numbers we try to raise rather than decrease in our bodies. However, pathogenic bacteria must be combated, and antibiotics are the primary weapons in this fight.

Synthetic antibiotics are antibiotics that are manufactured/formulated synthetically in pharmaceutical laboratories. Many people are unaware of the existence of antibiotics other than synthetic antibiotics. However, awareness of natural antibiotics is gradually spreading among the general public. Natural antibiotics differ from other forms of antibiotics in that they are "directly utilized by nature." They are not created in a laboratory. They are generally equally effective (if slightly slower to work) as antibiotics manufactured in pharmaceutical laboratories. Many people believe they are safer than antibiotics developed in laboratories.

One of the key reasons why everyone should have a basic understanding of natural antibiotics is to ensure that if you have a bacterial infection and don't have access to synthetically created antibiotics, you still have a way to treat the infection. This is significant since we know that some lethal bacterial infections are caused by this. And, while some activities can be completed on their own (such as the body's natural immune system), most will not be in remission on their own. In fact, when a bacterial disease emerges, it is assumed that the body's inherent immunity has already been overcome by germs. In this circumstance, unless something particularly catastrophic happens, the body is unlikely to recover the upper hand over microorganisms. The ailment in issue tends to worsen unless some kind of mitigating measures (such as an antibiotic) are taken.

As a result, within the context of "survivability," it would be beneficial for everyone to understand natural antibiotics so that they can distribute them in the event of a bacterial sickness where pharmaceutical antibiotics are unavailable. And, because the majority of the natural antibiotics we're talking about are plant parts that boost the body's immunity rather than directly kill bacteria, knowing about them (and then using them) would be a wise preventive practice.

Chapter 1: Synthetic Antibiotics vs. Natural Antibiotics

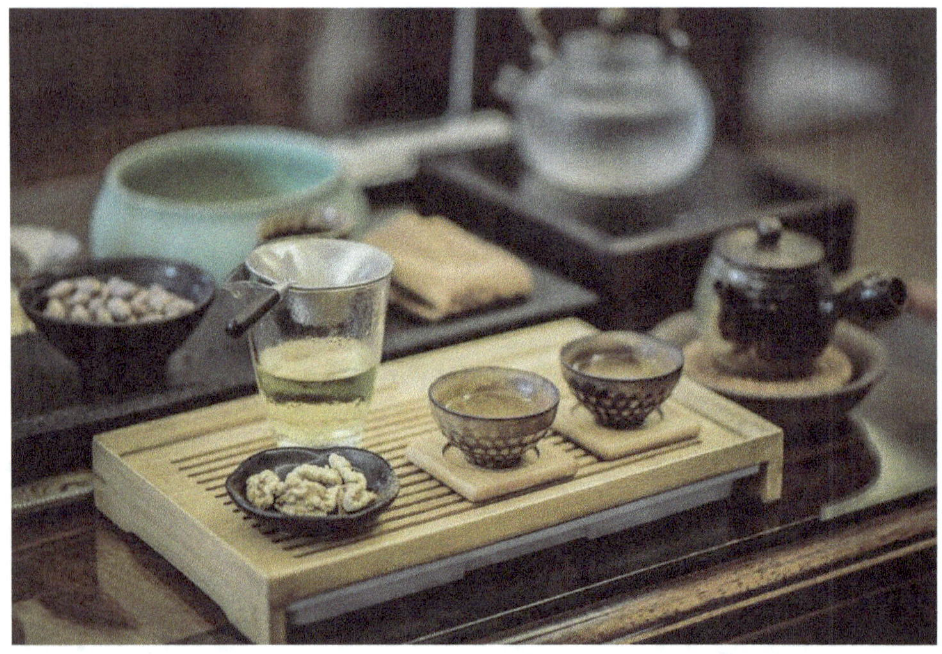

We can begin with descriptions, which both show chemicals known to aid in the battle against microorganisms that may try to damage us. The distinction between natural and manufactured antibiotics is that the former are non-toxic.

The former are natural products (directly exploited by the fields, common plant components), whereas the latter are laboratory-created chemical synthesis products. To create a synthetic antibiotic, you must first determine which chemical combinations have an antibiotic effect (that is, a bactericidal effect), then extract the compounds from the materials and combine them in the proper amounts to create the antibiotic. To obtain a natural antibiotic, on the other hand, you must first learn which plants (and which precise parts of them) have an antibiotic effect, and then go out into the fields to collect these parts of the plant, use them correctly, and benefit from the antibiotic effect. Of course, the distinction between natural antibiotics and synthetic supplements is not limited to definitions.

In terms of work speed, natural antibiotics differ from synthetic additives (typical). Synthetic antibiotics tend to be more effective than natural supplements. However, it is important to note that we are discussing typical scenarios here: because there are natural antibiotics that are proven to function faster than some synthetic medicines. However, the generally faster functioning speed connected with synthetic antibiotics is the major reason why synthetic supplements are commonly utilized in medical crises; when a person already suffers from an illness caused by a bacterial infection and immediate bacterial decimation is required. What is striking here is that the effectiveness of synthetic antibiotics tends to be their undoing, as most of them end up killing beneficial symbiotic bacteria unwittingly.

In terms of safety, natural supplements differ from synthetic antibiotics. Natural supplements are generally thought to be safer than synthetic antibiotics in many ways. It should be highlighted here that the usage of supplements is not always temporary (although it is ideal as it should be). On the contrary, some persons develop conditions that necessitate their use for an extended period of time or on a regular basis. If these people were to use synthetic antibiotics, they would very likely experience very unpleasant side effects as a result of the long-term usage of antibiotics. However, when gentler natural supplements are employed, the long-term prospects can be far better.

In terms of operating mechanisms, natural antibiotics differ from synthetic supplements (typical). We see a situation in which a conventional synthetic antibiotic operates by directly killing (killing) dangerous bacteria while also killing certain helpful bacteria. This is in contrast to the normal natural antibiotic, which works not only by killing germs but also by boosting the body's natural ability to fight future bacterial infections.

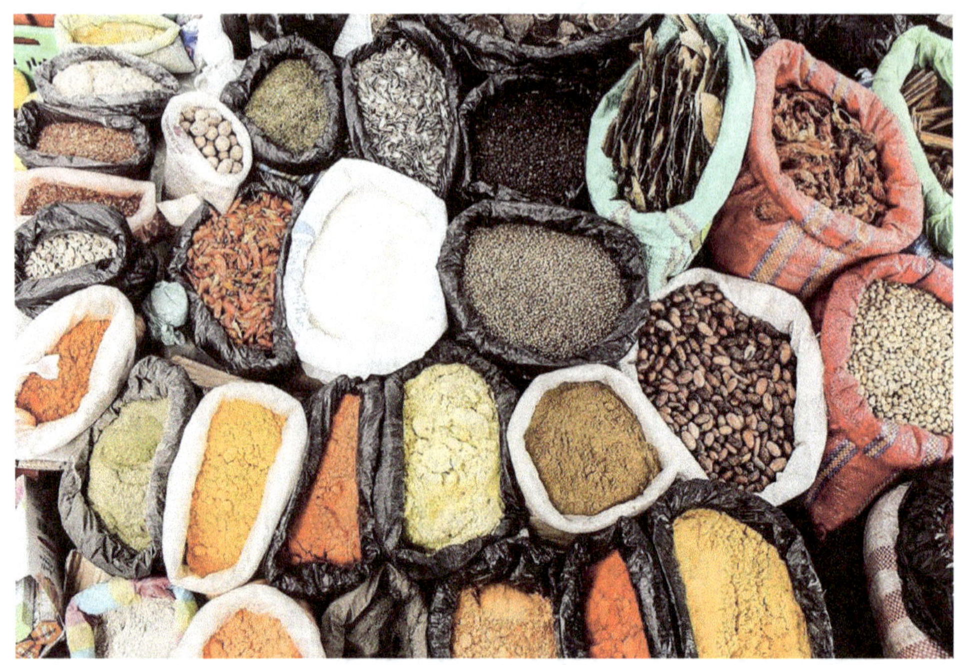

Why Are More People Turning to Natural Antibiotics?

In recent years, an increasing number of people have chosen to use natural antibiotics rather than the synthetic antibiotics that we once trusted. It's not as though natural (ancient) antibiotics are a brand-new innovation. These are substances that we have had since the beginning of time. These are the same medicines that our forefathers utilized to cure and prevent bacterial infections before the pharmaceutical business came along and offered us the most easily accessible synthetic antibiotics. As a result, they are not novel substances or discoveries. However, their extensive use in recent years is a new phenomena.

To have a context in which to understand, we must acknowledge that the human race as we know it now has lived for millions of years (according to scientific opinion), or at least thousands of years (according to most religious traditions). In both circumstances, it is undeniable that the human race has been around far longer than the pharmaceutical industry. Furthermore, there is little doubt that most of the microorganisms that are detrimental to us now were also hazardous to our forefathers. And it is in light of these facts that we have now realized that antibiotics are not a recent creation. They were always present; these are the ingredients that our forefathers utilized to treat the aforementioned antibacterial infections until the relatively recent birth of the pharmaceutical business.

Natural antibiotics were practically forgotten with the emergence of the pharmaceutical business. After all, the pharmaceutical business provided us with antibiotics that were both viciously effective and easily accessible (like pills that you could just pop and get almost instant relief).

This has been the case for many years, to the point where, as previously said, people have almost forgotten the natural antibiotics they took before to the entrance of those with synthetic formulas.

Then, only a few years ago, people began to reconsider natural medicines, and many began to utilize them instead of synthetic antibiotics. The reasons for this transition are of particular interest to us in our research.

Apparently, the most appealing aspect of natural antibiotics is their safety. For many years, there has been concern regarding the safety of synthetic antibiotics. Of course, they've always been brutally effective. However, it was also noted that their brutal effectiveness came at a high cost to those who employed it. Antibiotics would cause a slew of long-term negative effects. In an effort to assist us in eliminating harmful bacteria, most of them tended to eliminate beneficial bacteria in our bodies, leaving us with a new set of health issues. Furthermore, our bodies had a tendency to acquire resistance to them (after recognizing them for the "unnatural" foreign entities they were). This is essentially what drew people back to natural antibiotics, which are far safer (most of them are food items and plants that we already use on a daily basis, albeit for other reasons). Our bodies appear to be coping better with them. Natural antibiotics are also far less expensive than manufactured antibiotics.

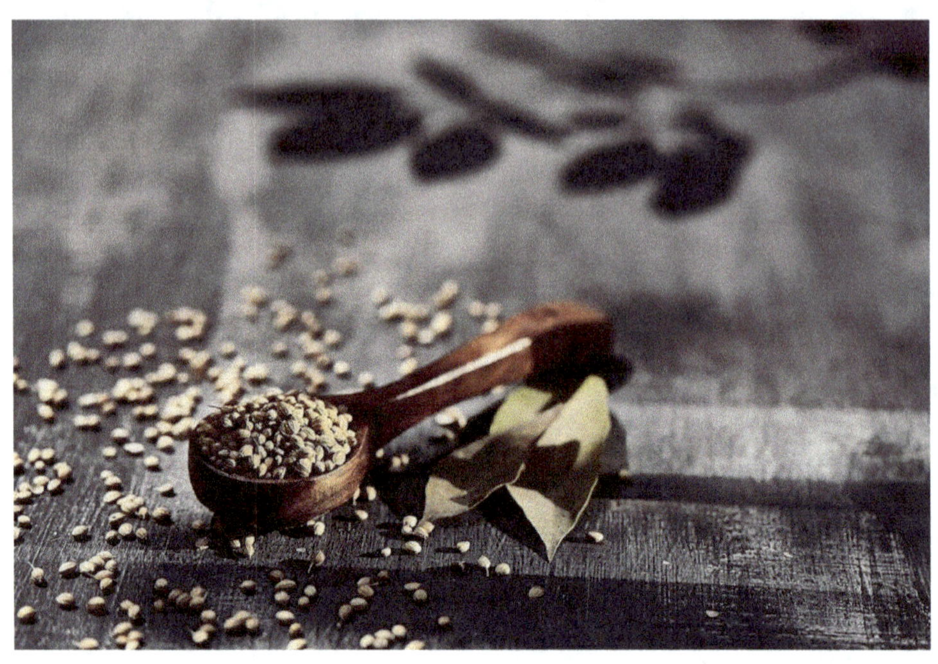

Natural Antibiotics' Two Primary Mechanisms of Action

Natural antibiotics act through two major processes. Before delving into the specifics of these two methods, it's a good idea to review the concept of antibiotics in general and natural antibiotics in particular. That would serve a number of objectives. It would be beneficial to the uninitiated (those of us who encounter these problems for the first time). This would provide a conceptual foundation for understanding the recently investigated working mechanisms.

Almost everything that kills bacteria is an antibiotic. This is one of the reasons why people want to destroy bacteria: when the bacteria become hazardous to their interests. Most of the time, we look at the microorganisms that cause our ailments. Bacterial infections create a wide range of diseases, some of which are mild and with which most of us live, while others are major illnesses (such as tuberculosis) that are lethal in nature. By extension, the term antibiotic may also apply to a medication that reduces the effects of harmful bacteria in the body, as well as a substance that increases the body's natural ability to combat bacteria. Because it was discovered that our bodies are continually in contact with hazardous bacteria, which we combat with antibiotics. However, unless our immunity is as robust as it should be, these germs are easily removed by our body naturally, without any assistance. However, sometimes our body's natural immunity is compromised, or we are exposed to a bacterial infection that we cannot avoid, and this results in disease, which is normally treatable with antibiotics.

Natural or synthetic antibiotics can be used. The first is an antibiotic produced "naturally," but the second is manufactured in a laboratory by combining Chemicals of various strengths. A typical natural antibiotic is a chemical derived from a plant portion.

As previously stated, these natural antibiotics function through two basic processes.

The first way by which natural antibiotics function is to actively kill offending bacteria. The antibiotic in question will simply be a lethal toxin for bacteria in this scenario. When you take a natural antibiotic, it finally makes its way into your bloodstream, where the offending bacteria will most likely have a field day." Bacteria eventually come into contact with it and perish as a result. The person is then cured of the condition that it created.

Natural antibiotics boost the body's ability to repel microorganisms through the second process. As previously said, when the bacterial population begins to grow to the point where it might cause disease, it is usually due to a failure of our body's natural immunity. In such circumstances, there is a potential to obtain greater (and more long-term) results by bolstering the body's natural ability to combat germs and other microbes that may try to damage you.

Bacterial Infection Treatment Suggestions:

Caffeine, alcohol, sugar, refined foods, meat, and dairy items should be avoided if suffering from an acute infection. Consume sparingly. Drink plenty of warm and atmospheric liquids, such as herbal tea. Fasting on juice or water for a few days can be quite beneficial during an infection. Enemas can aid in the rinsing of the system. Vitamin C, beta-carotene, and zinc are all indicated to help improve the immune system. Plants such as Echinacea and Hydrastis (Canadian hydrast) can assist support the immune system, although specific herbs are typically more beneficial. Saunas and steam baths can also help to detoxify the body during an infection. Massage, particularly foot massage with garlic oil, helps hasten the clearance of pollutants. Pay attention to what your body is attempting to tell you and inquire as to what it requires. Stay! When you're sick, don't push yourself past your boundaries. It is possible that recovery will take twice as long.

Throat Infection: Even if you have streptococcal angina (diagnosed by throat culture), natural therapies can be very helpful. However, it is important to check a blood test to ensure that no streptococci persist because an unnoticed streptococcal infection can occasionally lead to kidney, joint, or heart problems. Gargling with seawater, Calendula, Canadian Hydra, myrrh, or bitter orange oil can help with throat infections. There are numerous effective herbal medicines for the throat. Homeopathy is quite effective for throat infections. For sore throat, we frequently utilize Belladonna, Lachesis, Lycopodium, Phytolacca, and Mercurius. Streptococcal angina can also be treated with spigelia, a very unique medication that provides total pain relief in two days.

For bacterial skin infections, we use a combination of tincture and St. John's wort. Other herbs that are widely utilized include Canadian Hydra, comfrey, and plantain. Hot compresses, Ginger compresses, Epsom salt dips, and homeopathic treatments such as silica and Heparsulphuris can all be used to successfully cure bubbles and cysts. Fungal infections frequently react well to homeopathy or the use of diluted vinegar. Turmeric powder and tea oil can also help.

Bladder Infection: If you have a bladder infection, you should treat it right away. The longer you wait, the more discomfort you will experience, as well as an increased risk of kidney infection and the need for antibiotics. Water, cranberry juice or capsules, herbs (typically Hydrastis, bearberry, Bucchu, Chimaphilia, Berberis, and others), and homeopathy are all recommended (such remedies as Staphysagria, Cantharis, Apis, and Sarsaparilla, to name a few).
Remember, no dairy items if you have a breast infection! Consume plenty of hot ginger tea. We utilize an amazing Ayurvedic mixture called Sitopalades to break up the mucus. Kali bichromicum, Pulsatilla, Mercurius, Natrum muriaticum, and Allium cepa are effective homeopathic treatments.

Chapter 2: NATURAL ANTIBIOTICS AND PROBIOTICS

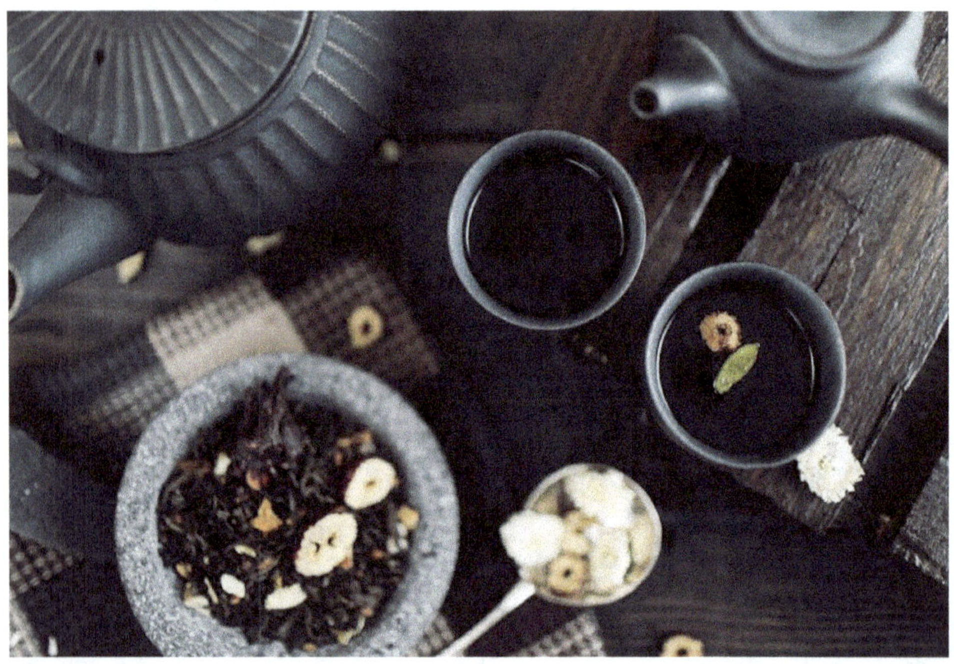

If you've ever been bitten by a wild animal, had a nasty wound, or been the unfortunate recipient of sexually transmitted illnesses, your friendly doctor will almost certainly prescribe antibiotics. Antibiotics are medications that either kill or slow the growth of microorganisms. Penicillin and amoxicillin are two antibiotics that are frequently administered.

The issue with synthetic antibiotics is that the human body can develop resistance to them. Every time you take antibiotics, your body develops a tolerance to them. As a result, using antibiotics for any ailment caused by bacteria reduces the body's ability to fight infections. The good news is that there are natural ways to avoid infection and enhance your immune system that does not need the use of these pharmaceuticals!

These antibacterial agents existed naturally in a range of foods and herbs long before Alexander Fleming, Nobel laureate and bacteriologist, identified them. Natural antibiotics and antibacterial compounds are mostly present in onion and garlic, herbs, honey, sauerkraut, and fermented foods including unpasteurized raw sauerkraut, raw pickles, and probiotic yogurt. All of these recipes boost the immune system and contain antibiotics. These meals encourage healthy digestion and aid in the defense of your body against infectious diseases.

Vitamin C-rich foods, such as cabbage, oranges and citrus fruits, tomatoes, papaya, sweet pepper, and kiwi, have powerful natural antibacterial and immunostimulant qualities. These fruits and vegetables are high in antioxidants, which protect cells from free radicals (unstable chemicals) that cause cancer.

Good microorganisms that aid digestion can be found in raw cabbage, raw cucumbers, and probiotic yogurt. This beneficial bacterium replaces harmful bacteria in the intestine, providing further protection against illness. A diet high in these items will help you battle bad germs and improve your overall health and well-being.
What about the onions and garlic you've requested? Sulfur compounds in onions and garlic have natural antimicrobial capabilities.

These substances act as anti-inflammatory agents and protect the body from colds and flu.
Natural antibacterial effects of honey were identified long before doctors developed prescribed drugs. Honey has a natural enzyme that causes the body to produce hydrogen peroxide. Hydrogen peroxide has the capacity to inhibit the

growth of many germs that could otherwise spread and cause disease.

Plants such as aloe, licorice, and practically all other herbs have antibacterial qualities that can aid in the battle against infections. Aloe vera gel is widely applied to cuts, burns, and other wounds to promote speedier healing and avoid bacterial infections. It's also effective against herpes simplex types 1 and 2. Licorice has antibacterial properties against streptococci, E. coli, staphylococcal infections, and even tuberculosis.

All of these natural antibiotics, if included in your everyday diet, will help you maintain a healthy immune system. Consuming these foods will help defend your body when it needs a little help fighting an army of microorganisms. So, the next time you get a cold, scratch your knee or engrave your hand on something, like a dinner pot, to acquire a natural antibiotic to help you heal quickly!

The Antibiotic and Antimicrobial Natural Wonder

We live in an era in which microorganisms are growing increasingly resistant to antibiotic treatment. Many of these illnesses, such as MRSA (methicillin-resistant Staphylococcus aureus), vancomycin-resistant worm or Enterococcus, and mycobacteria or tuberculosis, are deadly. The ability of a bacterium to resist the effects of antibiotics is referred to as resistance. This resistance occurs in nature as a result of natural selection, but it can also occur when "evolutionary" stress is applied to a specific population of bacteria, such as when antibiotic medication is overused or misused.

As a result, the number of organisms that have developed resistance to multiple antibiotics has increased. These are referred to as "super bacteria." Furthermore, the strongest antibiotics used to destroy these "super germs" can have unfavorable side effects on humans. In some situations, such as when treating a condition, these side effects might be hazardous. There is a remedy to the problem that contemporary medicine, particularly in the United States, has virtually completely overlooked. However, this option is gaining traction around the world, particularly in the holistic communities of Health and alternative medicine, as well as in countries with less bureaucracy to stifle the advancement of natural and non-pharmacological solutions. The use of the colloidal silver solution, a true natural antibiotic, is the solution.

The colloidal silver solution is a liquid suspension of small silver particles, colloidal particles that remain suspended without producing a dissolved or ionic solution. Colloidal silver is a well-known and potent antibacterial agent. Many infectious bacteria have been discovered to be killed at concentrations of five parts per million. It appears to work via the oligodynamic effect, suppressing the expression of enzymes and other proteins required for the production of ATP or adenosine-5'-triphosphate. It is poisonous to various resistant species, including MRSA and tuberculosis, and some recent research has revealed that it has an effect on viruses, including influenza A, the virus that causes influenza in humans.

Companies that manufacture or sell colloidal silver solutions in the United States are forbidden by the FDA from claiming any therapeutic value for the product. Even if it is a natural antibiotic, it cannot be branded as such. Until medication applications are submitted, the government authorizes you to label and sell them as a food supplement. Many independent laboratories are doing ongoing scientific studies to validate the effectiveness of this potential antibacterial Marvel, and colloidal silver has been tested with good results against various resistant and non-resistant diseases. In the United States, the EPA has approved its usage as a disinfectant in hospitals and medical clinics. Silver is also used to treat burns and bedsores.

However, the situation is radically different on a global scale. Many countries have recognized and utilized this potent substance, this natural antibiotic, to treat a variety of pathogenic diseases. The colloidal silver solution is widely used to treat malaria, cholera,

AIDS, influenza, hepatitis, respiratory infections such as pneumonia and bronchitis, tuberculosis, gonorrhea, sinus infections, food poisoning, vaginitis, staphylococcal infections and streptococci, Thrush, burns, wounds, and skin infections in African hospitals. It was effective against breast infections, peritoneal infections, oral infections, cuts, and wounds, according to the author.

This amazing metal appears to have no end to its wonderful effects. I recall the famous sculptor George Washington and his studies on peanuts. The colloidal silver solution could be the antibacterial miracle that the world sorely needs, as antibiotic-resistant super insects proliferate on a daily basis. We can only hope that American medicine will spread over the world and that colloidal money will be used to combat these enemies of our health. Please contact me if you want to learn more about this remarkable miraculous "metal," this potent natural antibiotic, or if you want to express your ideas, pro or con. I'd like to speak with you about this in person.

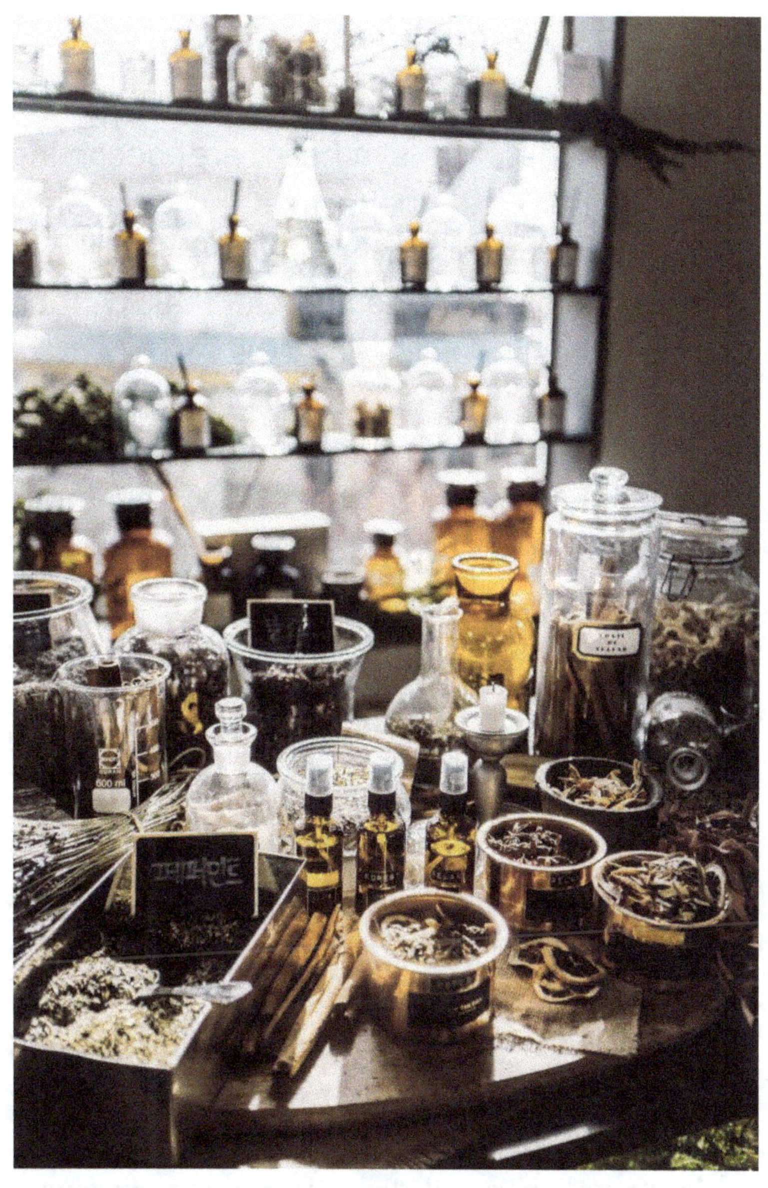

Synthetic Antibiotics' Adverse Effects

Antibiotics that are synthetic are becoming increasingly ineffective against microorganisms. However, antibiotics still have some unfavorable side effects that can be avoided by using antibiotic herbs.

1. **Infection of the Vaginal Yeast**

   As previously stated, the use of synthetic antibiotics effectively eliminates all "good" bacteria from the digestive tract. As healthy bacteria leave the gastrointestinal tract, yeast can start to grow by migrating into the vaginal and digestive Arena. This bacterial-yeast imbalance results in yeast infection. Yeast infection causes humiliating and unpleasant symptoms such as vaginal redness, swelling, itching, and burning. According to a 2013 antibiotic study, 25% of all women who took synthetic antibiotics had a yeast infection.

2. **Vomiting, nausea, and diarrhea**

   To establish good digestion, each digestive tract must maintain a healthy balance of good and bad bacteria. Synthetic antibiotics upset this balance, resulting in diarrhea.

According to a recent study, approximately 15% of all antibiotic users experience drug-related diarrhea.

3. Interaction of Drugs

The company's ongoing demand for more and more pharmaceuticals may result in drug interactions. Headache, stomach pain, and other major health problems can occur as a result of these interactions. Furthermore, other synthetic antibiotics can significantly impair the body's capacity to function normally. The usage of some oral contraceptives is one example. Other synthetic antibiotics can interfere with contraception and result in an unintended pregnancy. To guarantee effective functioning, patients must maintain regular communication with doctors regarding the drugs they consume.

4. Induced allergens or hypersensitivity

Several patients have reported allergic reactions to synthetic medications. Antibiotics were responsible for approximately 32% of cases of medication allergy, according to a 2011 study. These allergens are visibly visible on the skin, causing rashes or urticaria.

Other uncommon adverse effects include kidney stones, light sensitivity, hearing loss, and infrequent abnormalities in blood coagulation.

The present synthetic antibiotic dilemma
The media accused him of being the source of all the speakers. The world is experiencing an antibiotic crisis. Bacteria are becoming increasingly resistant to the synthetic antibiotics that doctors use, resulting in the latest bacterial outbreak. New synthetic medications must be produced to compete with each new bacterium that emerges. How is this feasible in such a short period of time? Bacteria are, in essence, among the most adaptive organisms on the earth. They reproduce in twenty minutes, whereas humans often wait twenty years before reproducing. Furthermore, each reproduction results in a new evolution. These new bacterium strains can also instruct other bacteria strains on how to build against other strains. And how long can it continue? The medical community recognizes that the era of synthetic antibiotics is coming to an end. People must begin preparing for an unexpected future.

For numerous years, doctors overused and over-diagnosed allegedly "miraculous" medications, which contributed to the antibiotic crisis. Penicillin, the amazing drug that wiped out innumerable ailments in the mid-twentieth century, is a prime example of this overdiagnosis. It was developed in 1942, but forty million pounds of penicillin were used in the United States each year less than half a century later.

Today, more than sixty million pounds of penicillin are used each year, with the drug eventually becoming obsolete in the next century owing to overuse. As previously stated, bacteria can be engineered to resist the onslaught of antibiotics. Because microorganisms are resistant to penicillin, the overuse of the medicine will most likely result in a disaster.

Furthermore, studies reveal that synthetic antibiotics enter and leave the body relatively unchanged. This means that they work their way through the digestive system, as well as in the world's largest "water," without affecting it. Even after the water has been cleansed by underground processes, it still has low quantities of this antibiotic "rejection." As a result, even if people drink tap water, they develop a minor tolerance to toothier antibiotics. Finally, these medicines will not be effective on these people because the germs in their bodies already know how to fight them.

Of course, reducing the usage of synthetic antibiotics in today's culture is challenging due to societal thinking. Who can blame people for wanting to get rid of their diseases as soon as possible? Nobody likes to feel bad. Nobody wants to die as a result of the disease. Because they work immediately, synthetic antibiotics are invaluable. They are extremely effective in all life-threatening disease scenarios. However, society must limit the use of synthetic antibiotics and save them from life-threatening situations. It is vital to limit the antibiotics used in the current environmental onslaught, as a result of the water supply. Furthermore, the use of these antibiotics should be reduced in order to improve the vigor and health of farm animals. Synthetic antibiotics serve a purpose and were developed for a specific cause. However, these justifications have been broadened to cover practically the entire globe, rendering them almost obsolete in the coming years.

Furthermore, with each dose of synthetic antibiotics, people's immune systems quickly begin to deteriorate. The immune system is an incredible mechanism that first permits a person to steadily repel bacterial invasions. Synthetic antibiotics, on the other hand, permeate the body and destroy both beneficial and bad germs. They, for example, eliminate the undeniably crucial flora of the digestive tract. This eradication of flora might result in yeast infections and unpleasant stomach symptoms. Remember that the body requires ongoing defense against persistent attacks, and removing these helpful bacteria first produces a tasteless environment in which you can quickly grow worse.

People must adhere to a specified "course" when using synthetic antibiotics. When a person begins an antibiotic but does not finish the prescribed course, he or she leaves live heavy bacteria in his or her system. This remaining bacteria is actively working to regenerate the "next generation" of surviving bacteria, allowing them to develop resistance to the very drugs that may have killed them.

The antibiotic problem has resulted in a vicious spiral of harsher medications, stronger bacteria, and weaker immune systems. People must begin to focus on the eventual benefits of utilizing herbal antibiotics in order to break the cycle and feed towards improved overall health.

Natural Antiviral Herbs That Are Common

There are hundreds of herbs that have been shown to have considerable antiviral action when taken. Some are easy to find in your garden or at the local market, while others are more difficult to find. It is best to consult a herbal product expert to determine the proper dosage and circumstances of use. Some plants, for example, should not be consumed when pregnant. Also, keep in mind that the majority of the herbs listed are used to treat more than one viral infection. Some are also powerful enough to eliminate all other hazardous viruses. It's also conceivable to come into an infection that has more than one natural cure.

Olive leaf can be taken as a capsule or as tea with mint. It is most commonly used to treat influenza, colds, and herpes.
Another herb with antiviral effects is balm on lemon leaves. When used locally, it is used to treat stomach disorders and skin infections. An infusion can be prepared for oral administration (add warm water). It is thought that it is not safe to use during pregnancy.

Adding ginger to tea and meals not only makes them taste better but is also believed to help prevent and shorten the duration of colds. It also reduces neck and chest pain. It is a powerful herb in the treatment of influenza and the relief of sore throat when combined with honey. It can also be crushed or sliced into little pieces before being mixed with hot water.

Chlorella is a small unicellular green alga that is not just high in nutrients but also known to boost the immune system. A healthy immune system aids in the battle against viruses, avoiding infection or the spread of infection.

Chamomiles are used in the preparation of herbal infusions for medicinal purposes. This daisy-like plant is used to treat gastrointestinal issues, as well as to alleviate inflammation and ulcers. The removal of crushed juice, which is put to hot water, is preferred.

Cayenne pepper is without a doubt one of the most potent herbs on the planet. It has numerous medical characteristics, including the treatment and relief of colds, sore throats, and stomach ache, as well as the prevention of the emergence of other diseases such as fungi. It is used as a spice in meals.

Cranberry is utilized for more than just cooking; it is also a powerful medicinal plant. It is used to treat gastrointestinal issues as well as circulatory difficulties. A full or half-full cup of fruit juice is consumed. Because it is sweet, you do not need to add sweetness, as you would with other herbs.

The weed, also known as black-bunched Acea, is often used to treat kidney infections and sore throats. For a few days, the grass is pressed and drunk to see how it affects the body. However, the herb might cause dizziness, headaches, cramps, nausea, vomiting, sweating, and low blood pressure.

For millennia, chili has been utilized in traditional medicine, particularly in Asian nations such as India. It is employed in the treatment of herpes and other respiratory diseases. It is one of the most extensively used spices in the world and is used in cuisine or locally by adding water or milk.

Garlic is a proven traditional medication. It is used to treat a variety of ailments, including warts, influenza, and colds. There are additional natural ways to treat genital warts, such as taking oat showers or applying onion slices to warts. However, the onion has not been scientifically confirmed. I recommend that you see a doctor because these medications only cure warts and not the HPV that causes warts. Chewing raw garlic is said to treat patients with high blood pressure. Garlic is commonly used in cooking, despite the fact that it has a strong odor that does not go away easily.

Astragalus Root is utilized as an anti-influenza treatment. It works best by boosting the body's immune system, allowing it to fight pathogens. It is advised to utilize it prior to the flu season, rather than when you already have it. Use it in herbal teas or prepared dishes.

Cat bile is a powerful antiviral, antibacterial, and antifungal herb that can be taken as a pill or as a tea. It is also a potent immune system stimulator.

We can't discuss herbs without including aloe vera. It is a plant that can treat practically every ailment. It belongs to the same family as the agave. It is very harsh and may require additional sweetener; honey is preferred. It is quite effective and can be taken orally or locally.

Elderberry tree roots, leaves, seeds, and berries are used to treat colds and flu. Because of the high content of cyanide in the plant, it must be fully boiled before being used as a medicine.

Oregano oil is used as a medication as well as a flavoring agent in cuisine. When used topically, it is a potent antiviral since it speeds up the healing process and prevents skin irritation.

In the treatment of stomach ulcers, licorice root is used as a tea that can be drunk alone or combined with other herbal teas. It has antibacterial and antiviral properties.

The majority of bacteria found in the human body are not hazardous; in fact, they are extremely useful. Only 1% of the bacteria in our bodies are thought to be dangerous. The remainder is beneficial to digestion and other vital bodily functions. Some bacteria are also known to reduce the incidence of cancer and to aid in the respiratory and urinary tracts.

Bacteria, unlike viruses, are living microorganisms that can live and multiply without being attached to a living cell. They are also more massive than viruses.

Bacterial Infections That Are Common

It is well understood that not all bacteria are innocuous and beneficial; others are extremely dangerous and can have a substantial impact on human health. Tuberculosis is one of these infections that affects millions of individuals, particularly in Sub-Saharan Africa. It is highly contagious and widely dispersed in the air. It affects the respiratory system, especially the lungs, and if not recognized and treated promptly, it can be fatal.

Typhoid, tetanus, syphilis, pneumonia, Hansen's disease, cavities, gingivitis, epiglottitis, Tonsillitis, Legionnaires disease, whooping cough, anthrax, and meningitis are among the other prevalent bacterial infections. Bacteria can be transferred through unprotected sexual contact. Syphilis, chlamydia, and gonorrhea are among them. These infections can be cured. Other consequences, such as pelvic inflammatory disease, should be detected and treated as soon as possible.

Prostatitis is a bacterial infection that affects men's prostates. Some bacteria can cause urinary tract infections in women.

Home natural antibiotics

Antibiotics are also known as antibacterial medications. Pharmaceutical antibiotics are derived from fungus. They are employed in the treatment and treatment of bacterial infections. Antibiotic abusers are known to develop resistance, which means that drugs cannot be administered.

Most pharmaceutical antibiotics recommended by doctors may produce side effects such as nausea, dizziness, and vomiting, while others may induce allergic reactions such as skin rash or itching; still, others may destroy the good bacteria that aid in some of the body's processes. When taking natural substances, we cannot rule out the possibility of side effects; nevertheless, if any and all of them are manageable, there are fewer side effects.

Millions of people are allergic to specific herbs; some are sensitive to nuts, some to honey, and still others to berries. One of the benefits of adopting natural therapies is that they are common to look for more than one natural remedy for infection. In this instance, you have the option of picking one; you are not allergic. Let's take a look at some common natural antibiotics and infections that can be treated.
Garlic and onions have been utilized for centuries for their antibacterial and antiviral properties. They believe they help lower inflammation and the risk of hypertension and stroke.

Any diet high in vitamin C has been shown to have antibacterial and antiviral effects. They boost the body's immunity, allowing it to protect itself and heal more quickly. Fruits and vegetables rich in vitamin C include strawberries, lemons and limes, pineapple, melons, and oranges, as well as broccoli, tomatoes, spinach, cabbage, and cabbage. Not only is kiwi high in vitamin C, but it should also be high in all other vital elements. It is the most nutrient-dense fruit, but it is also one of the most expensive.

Eucalyptus contains a potent antiseptic that destroys the majority of infections, including bacteria. It is mixed into tea and adds a lovely flavor.

Some germs are passed on to us through the food we eat. The inclusion of horseradish in one's diet. Bacteria are killed even before entering the body. It's eaten as a vegetable. Lauric acid, which is found in coconut oil, is an important chemical. Its primary purpose is to disintegrate pathogens. Oil can be used in the production of foods or consumed on its own.

Fermented foods, such as fermented vegetables, have been suggested by scientists as a way to assist the body to receive the correct microorganisms. These foods are known as probiotics, and they are advised for usage in conjunction with antibiotics.

Marshmallow root is reported to have analgesic effects. It can also be used to destroy bacteria in the urinary tract. It is better to take it orally as an infusion (with warm water). Yarrow is another herb that can be used to treat urinary tract infections. It is also used to make tea. It is not advised to use it when pregnant because it can trigger uterine contractions.

Turmeric is a powerful medicinal herb that is typically processed into a yellow/orange powder. It is used to treat bacterial, fungal, and viral infections, among others.

Chapter 3: HERBAL REMEDIES ARE POWERFUL ANTIBIOTICS

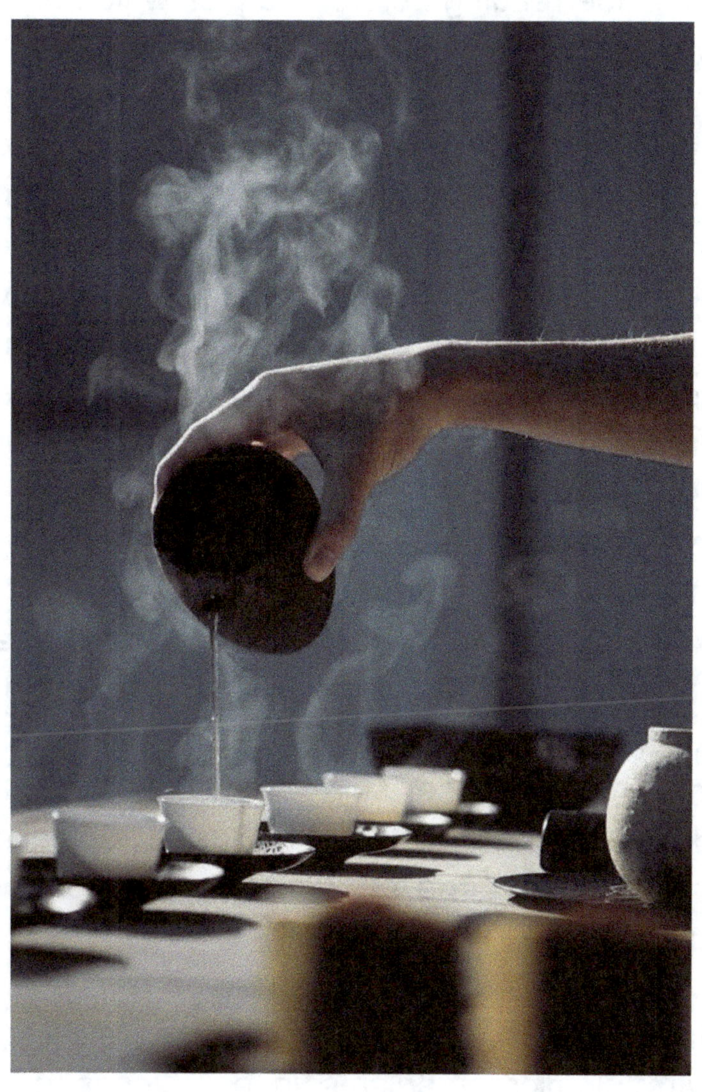

Do you take this medication if you are very ill? Do you intend to use natural remedies? Or are you going to opt for pharmaceutical drugs? Continue reading before you pick which of the two possibilities is best for you.

When comparing the efficacy of herbal medicines with pharmaceutical drugs, we question which is the most potent. Some people are skeptical about herbal therapies because they believe plants are less effective than medications. Herbalists responded that herbs are natural gifts to mankind. God created nature, hence herbal treatments were developed by God. So, who do you believe is the more powerful? Is it the work of God or of man?

Antibiotics have been recognized as humanity's "biggest breakthrough" in medicine. Antibiotics are used to kill bacteria or germs that may be the source of our ailments. However, the majority of the human population is unaware of the hazardous side effects of antibiotics.

Yes, antibiotics can kill both beneficial and dangerous microorganisms. They eliminate harmful microorganisms in our bloodstream.

The bad news is that even good bacteria, such as white flakes, die. After seven days of medication, there are still nasty bacteria inside us that can multiply in great numbers and quickly become dangerous germs that might cause serious harm. We become sad, weary, and more susceptible to respiratory infections. According to recent research, prescription medications have more heinous side effects than alternative therapies.

According to the study, Paxil should not be administered to individuals who have suicidal tendencies because it will only make the patient's condition worse. Viagra is also on the list of medications that have negative side effects. The origins of blindness.

It is possible that taking acidophilus after taking antibiotics suggested by your doctor is a good idea. Acidophilus capsules are said to contain billions of beneficial bacteria. Yogurt and grapefruit seed extract pills are also good sources of acidophilus. Take, most significantly, oregano.

Herbalists contend that oregano is nature's most potent antibiotic. Oregano, as an effective herbal medicine, has been clinically demonstrated to eradicate harmful germs that even the most potent antibiotics cannot eliminate. Oregano is available in the form of oil or pills. This can be taken orally or in combination with grapefruit juice.

Another essential property of oregano is that it promotes the growth of white flakes while killing black weeds.

Oregano relieves sinusitis, asthma, bronchitis, emphysema, and other respiratory disorders or allergies when taken on a daily basis.
So it's entirely up to you. Regardless of the drug, remember that your acts and the consequences of those actions are entirely your responsibility. Check that these do not jeopardize other people or yourself—prevention is better than treatment.

RESISTANCE TO ANTIBIOTICS

Antibiotic resistance is a type of medication resistance that occurs when bacteria survive after being exposed to one or more antibiotics. These are referred to as "multi drug resistant" (MDR) or, more colloquially, "superbugs."

MRSA is the most well-known of these superbugs (methicillin-resistant Staphylococcus aureus).

Superbug drug resistance can be caused by mutation or the acquisition of resistant genes from other bacteria. It can, however, be blamed on the widespread usage of antibiotics. They have become so adapted to our bodies that they no longer have the desired effect on our immune system.

AMR stands for antimicrobial resistance.

The World Health Organization made the following recommendations on how to tackle antibiotic resistance on April 30, 2018:
Antibiotics should only be taken if prescribed by a doctor. Even if you feel better, finish the complete course of antibiotics.
Never give antibiotics to others or use leftover recipes.

While drug overuse is a contributing contributor to antibiotic resistance, there are other things you can do every day to prevent it.

Wash your hands before and after handling meals, use the restroom, and change diapers. When coughing or sneezing, cover your mouth and nose.

Blowing and cleaning the nose using tissues, then removing them correctly. I'm not a spitter. Stay at home if you are sick. If you continue to feel poorly after taking antibiotics, see your doctor.

The number of diseases designated as "superbugs" grows over time, however, for the time being, the following list is relevant:

Staphylococcus aureus - MRSA) - found on mucosal membranes and human skin, MRSA was one of the first germs to show penicillin resistance in 1947. This disease is exceedingly frequent and is responsible for many hospital deaths.
Streptococcus and Enterococcus require a mix of medications to be eradicated. Pneumonia, bacteremia, otitis media, meningitis, sinusitis, peritonitis, and arthritis are all caused by Streptococcus.

Pseudomonas aeruginosa is a common opportunistic infection. Antibiotics have little effect on it.

Clostridium nosocomial bacterium causes diarrhea in hospitals worldwide. According to several studies, Clostridium Colitis is induced by the overuse of antibiotics in animals.
Salmonella and E. coli are frequently the result of consuming contaminated water. Because of the increasing usage of antibiotics, they grew more harmful, with more deaths.

Acinetobacter Baumannii-5. In November 2004, the Centers for Disease Control and Prevention (CDC) stated that an increasing number of persons had Acinetobacter in medical devices or soldiers who have fought in Iraq or Kuwait.

Klebsiella Pneumoniae is a new gram-negative Bacillus that is highly resistant to treatments and causes infections with significant morbidity and mortality in a number of clinical settings around the world.

Mycobacterium Tuberculosis-multidrug-resistant tuberculosis kills 150,000 people each year. This was exacerbated by an upsurge in the HIV/AIDS epidemic. Tuberculosis was one of the most common diseases, and there was no cure until Selman Waksman discovered streptomycin in 1943. Bacteria, on the other hand, quickly evolved resistance. Drugs such as isoniazid and rifampicin have been utilized since then. Drug resistance arises in Mycobacterium Tuberculosis through spontaneous mutations in its genomes.

In humans, Neisseria Gonorrhoeae is a sexually transmitted pathogen that can cause pelvic pain, urine pain, penile and vaginal discharge, as well as systemic symptoms. The bacterium was first detected in 1879, according to records. Penicillin treatment was effective for 40 years, but by 70 years, a drug-resistant strain had emerged.

These superbugs are frequently treated with a cocktail of potent antibiotics. Experts and scientists are continuously looking for weaknesses in these viruses in order to give them a better chance of defeating them.

Here is an important comment from one of the scientists who have committed their lives to this cause. "The discovery of a fungus capable of rendering these multidrug-resistant germs incapable of further infection is huge," says Irena Kenneley, a microbiologist and infectious disease specialist at Case Western Reserve University's Frances Payne Bolton School of Nursing in Cleveland. "More treatment alternatives will save many more lives in the long run." Because the use of antibiotics in agriculture (which encourages growth and prevents infection in animals) has led to the mutation of resistant diseases, one method to increase the chances is to consume only meat raised on organic farms.

There are other, more natural ways to assist your immune system in combat harmful bacteria, which include:

Tea tree oil has been shown to combat and kill staphylococcal germs. It is applied directly to the affected skin as a topical application.

Apple cider vinegar and baking soda—by combining these two ingredients, you can create a paste that functions similarly to tea tree oil.

Garlic-a complex garlic composition is great for activating the immune system and combating illnesses.

Coriander oil - According to a 2011 study undertaken by Portuguese researchers, coriander oil is effective against 12 deadly germs.

Pascalite is a kind of bentonite clay found solely in the Wyoming highlands. Its tendency to promote wound infections when used locally within a few hours or days, resulting in complete recovery.

Turmeric is a medicinal herb that has been used for ages to treat bacterial and viral diseases. Anti-inflammatory and antibacterial activities have been demonstrated.

Honey Makuna, when combined with turmeric, is an effective treatment for MRSA and other superbugs.

Oregano oil has been shown to be effective in fighting bacteria and staphylococcal infections. Olive leaf extract includes an active component that helps the immune system fight illnesses that are resistant to medications.

Echinacea is mostly used to cure colds and flu, but it has also been used to treat open wounds, diphtheria, cellulitis, blood poisoning, syphilitic sores, and other bacterial infections in the past. It has the capacity to eliminate even the most difficult bacteria.

Colloidal silver-germicides and antibacterial capabilities were identified about a century ago. Numerous clinical instances and anecdotal data indicate that colloidal silver can destroy germs, fungi, and viruses.
Pau d'arco is a South American plant whose active ingredient order has been shown to cure a wide range of diseases, including those caused by bacteria, viruses, and fungus.
So, while there are presently no recognized cures for these superbugs, there are things we can do to protect ourselves and aid in the fight against these bacteria using traditional and herbal medicines.

Everything You Need to Know About Antibiotics

The decision to use natural antibiotics is entirely personal. As stated in the previous chapter, all information is essential for changing one's way of life when using herbal medicines, including antibiotics. You must ensure that they are appropriate for you. Of course, in an emergency case, such as a severe illness or trauma can cause standard antibiotics to function. Herbal treatments perform best for preventive, chronic diseases, and the side effects of antibiotics.

According to the findings of this study, about one-third of all Americans utilize herbal treatments. Although there are several things you can do to ensure that they are safe for you and your health:

Other medications you are taking - you will need to consult your doctor to ensure that they are not acting abnormally.

Side effects - Although herbal medicines have far fewer side effects than conventional antibiotics, you should always be aware of what options are available if they are assigned. Herbal therapies are not regulated as complementary treatment. There are numerous tools and information available to assist you in making your decision, however, some organizations have not been sufficiently evaluated on pregnant or nursing women, children, or the elderly.

Infection can be divided into two categories: heat and wetness." This shows that antibiotics are excellent for treating "hot" as part of the infection-fever, sore throat, inflammation-due to the fact that they frequently leave the symptoms of "wet" – mucus, nausea, foggy head-the only one.

As a result, many herbalists frequently propose combining herbal treatment with conventional medicine.

Antibiotics are mostly used to treat bacterial infections, such as moderate acne, which is not very severe but is unlikely to be resolved without the use of antibiotics.

Conditions that are not particularly harmful but have the potential to spread to others if not treated promptly, such as the skin infection impetigo or the sexually transmitted infection Chlamydia.

Conditions, such as kidney illness, where data suggests that antibiotics could greatly hasten to heal.

Cellulite and pneumonia are examples of conditions that can lead to more serious problems.

The development of antibiotics began in 1877 when Louis Pasteur discovered that saprophytic bacteria might suppress the growth of the germs responsible for the sickness. Then, in 1928, Alexander Flemming made the discovery that led to penicillin, which was the most significant contribution to the field of antibiotics. Since the 1970s, to be exact. For many years, the majority of novel antibiotics were synthetic adaptations of natural antibiotics.

Fermentation is the method by which antibiotics are created. If you're interested in participating in this process, the processes are as follows:

1. Before fermentation begins, the bacterium that produces the essential antibiotics should be identified and multiplied numerous times. A beginning culture is generated in the laboratory using a sample of previously separated and chilled organisms for this purpose. When establishing the initial culture, a sample of the organism is introduced to an Agar plate. The initial culture is then placed in bottles with a mixture of food and other nutrients required for growth. This results in a suspension that can be transported to growth reservoirs.

2. Seed tanks are steel tanks that are meant to create an ideal environment for microorganism growth. They contain everything a specific bacterium would require to exist and thrive, such as hot water meals and carbohydrates like lactose or glucose sugar. They also contain other required carbon sources, such as acetic acid, alcohols, or hydrocarbons, as well as

nitrogen sources, such as ammonia salts. Growth elements such as vitamins, amino acids, and micronutrients surround the makeup of the tray's seeds. Tank seeds have mixers to keep the growth media flowing and a pump to assure sterilized and filtered air. The material in the tanks is moved to the primary tanks for fermentation after around 24-28 hours.

3. The fermentation tank is essentially a larger version of the steel seed tank, which can store approximately 30,000 gallons. It is stuffed with the same growth media housed in a seed tank, which also provides an inductive development environment. Microorganisms can thrive and multiply in this environment. They secrete a huge amount of the desired antibiotic throughout this procedure. The tanks must be chilled to a temperature between 23 and 27 degrees Fahrenheit (73 and 81 degrees Celsius). 2 degrees Celsius). A steady stream of sterilized air flows out while the container is constantly stirred. As a result, anti-foaming chemicals are frequently included. Because pH regulation is required for optimal growth,

they provide the necessary acid or base to the reservoir.

4. After three to five days, the maximum number of antibiotics has been generated, and the isolation procedure can begin. The fermentation broth is cleaned using a variety of procedures depending on the antibiotic generated. For example, the ion exchange approach can be used to purify water-soluble antibiotic drugs. The component is removed from the organic waste in the broth and transported to a device that separates other essential water-soluble compounds throughout this process. A solvent extraction method is used to isolate an oil-soluble antibiotic, such as penicillin. In this procedure, the broth is treated with organic solvents that can particularly dissolve the antibiotic, such as butyl acetate or methylisobutyl ketone. The dissolved antibiotic is subsequently produced using a variety of organic chemical methods. Manufacturers typically leave a pure powder form of the antibiotic at the end of this process, which can be refined into various sorts of goods.

5. Antibiotics come in a variety of forms. It can be purchased in tablet or gel capsule form for intravenous bags or syringes, or it can be purchased in powder form for incorporation into topical ointments. Following the initial isolation, many rounds of refining can take place, depending on the ultimate form of the antibiotic. Crystalline antibiotics can be dissolved in IV bag solution and placed in a bag, which is then tightly closed. The antibiotic tablet physically fills the bottom half of the gel capsule, while the upper half is mechanically put. The antibiotic is added into the ointment when used in local ointments.

6. The antibiotic is now being transferred to the final packing station. The products are stored and packed in boxes here. They are placed onto vehicles and sent to wholesalers, hospitals, and pharmacies. The entire fermentation, recovery, and treatment procedure might take anywhere from five to eight days.

This antibiotic works by exploiting the structural differences between bacterial cells and host cells. They prevent bacterial cell multiplication, keeping their number constant, letting the body combat bacteria with natural defenses or fully kill them.

These antibiotics can be given in three different ways:

Orally-tablets, pills, and capsules, as well as a liquid to drink, can be used to treat the majority of mild to moderately severe infections in the body.
Topical creams, creams, sprays, or drops are frequently used to treat skin infections.
Injections - These injections are normally reserved for more serious infections and can be given as injections or drip infusions directly into the blood or into the muscle.
Synthetic antibiotics are classified into six groups:
Penicillins are commonly used to treat infections such as skin infections, chest infections, and urinary tract infections.

Cephalosporins are effective in treating a wide spectrum of diseases, but they are especially effective in treating more serious illnesses including septicemia and meningitis. Because aminoglycosides can have major side effects such as hearing loss and renal damage, they are only used to treat very serious conditions such as sepsis. They swiftly break down inside the digestive system, necessitating injection. They are also used as drops to treat some ear and eye infections.

Tetracyclines are antibiotics that can be used to treat a variety of ailments. They are often used to treat moderate to severe acne, as well as rosacea, a skin condition that causes redness and patches.

Macrolides are particularly effective in the treatment of pulmonary and thoracic infections. They can also be used to treat penicillin-resistant germs or to treat persons who are allergic to penicillin.
Fluoroquinolones are antibiotics with a broad spectrum of action that can be used to treat a variety of infections.
But, what exactly were natural antibiotics? How can you know which ones are best for you? No, there are other sources of information available, with a doctor or pharmacist being one of them. You can, of course, try to

persuade them to stick with traditional treatment, but if you stick to your guns, they will be extremely useful in what they can and cannot accept due to the present prescription list. Of course, the greatest thing you can do is try to decide whether herbal medicines are suited for you as soon as I couldn't find anywhere that they are safe for you to take. You'll know how effective it is for your body once you've tried the appropriate dose.

In many situations, experts are unsure which chemical in a single herb acts to treat sickness or illness. Whole herbs contain a variety of chemicals that, when combined, can have a positive effect. Many things have contributed to efficacy. The type of environment (temperature, bugs, soil quality, etc.) in which the plant grows, for example, will influence how and when it is picked and processed.

Natural antibiotics operate in two ways: they kill hazardous germs and boost the body's natural defenses. Many foods, beverages, and seasonings provide the required natural antibacterial characteristics.

The following are some examples, along with information on how they work:

Oil of Oregano

There are numerous components and foods that have natural antibacterial action. For example, oregano oil is high in thymol and carvacrol, two powerful antibacterial and antifungal chemicals. They can aid in the prevention of subsequent bacterial infections. In comparison to other antimicrobial oils, oregano essential oil is particularly effective against a variety of bacteria. According to research, it is an effective antibiotic against Staphylococcus aureus (staphylococcus).

Oregano oil has been shown to be effective in the treatment of respiratory tract infections, gastrointestinal issues, menstrual cramps, and urinary tract infections. It can also be used locally to treat skin issues such as acne and dandruff.

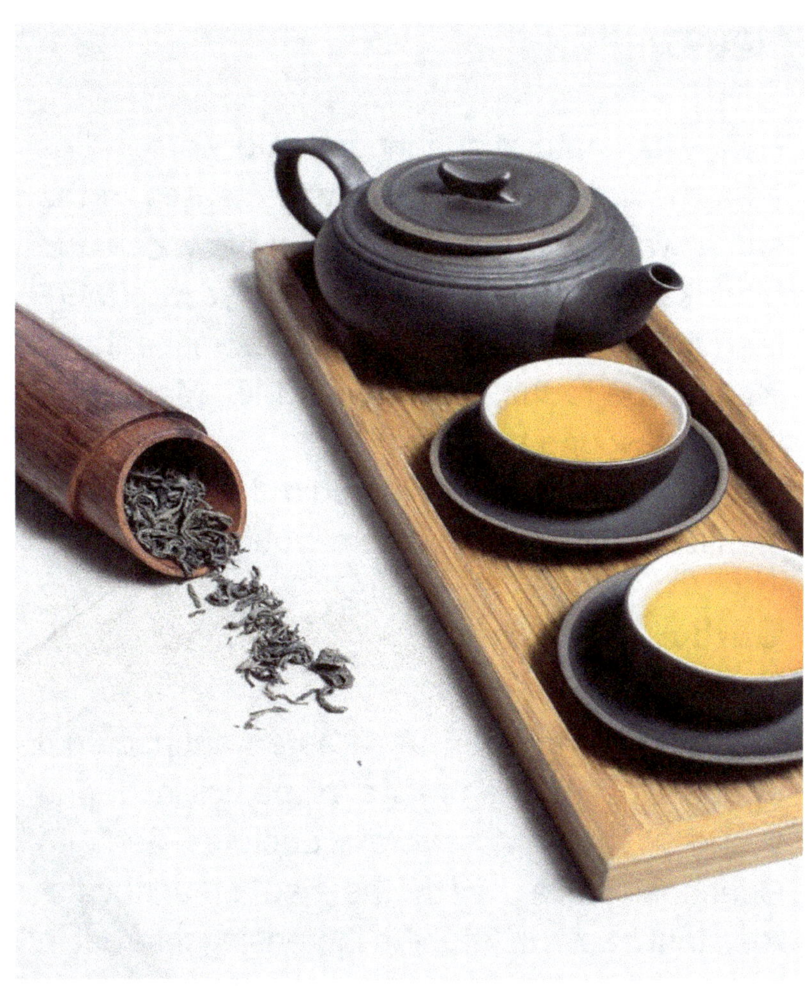

Honey

Honey has natural anti-inflammatory properties as a meal, but not all honey is created in the same way. Other ingredients in New Zealand Manuka honey include methylglyoxal (MG). Manuka honey is thought to have antibacterial effects due to the presence of MG. Manuka is ideal for wound healing.

It is, however, a honey medic that has been sterilized and marketed as a wound bandage.

Garlic

Garlic has long been used as an antibacterial agent. Due to a shortage of penicillin during World War II, several doctors fled to Czechoslovakia. "With the rise of antibiotic-resistant bacteria, there is increasing interest in the study of garlic's active component.

Because allicin degrades under heat, it must be consumed raw. Crude Czech oil can also be used as a local antibacterial agent "McCrae says. Garlic has been used to treat colds and flu, fungal infections, warts, and hypertension, and it may have potential in major conditions like diabetes, heart disease, and some malignancies.

Tea Tree Essential Oil

Tea tree oil is antiseptic and effective against some bacteria strains. The oil of the Melaleuca tree species has been shown to be the most effective and least irritating to the skin. Tea tree oil is used to treat skin conditions such as acne, fungal infections, and athlete's foot, as well as vaginal infection, oral herpes, and ear infections.

Elderberry Joy

A number of recent studies have highlighted the immune-boosting properties of elderberry water-based extracts and juice, as well as free radical scavenging activity, which can protect cells from damage, infection, and disease. Almonds, blueberries, and blackberries were used to treat influenza, cough, colds, and intent. Their antioxidant properties may also aid in the reduction of bad cholesterol and the prevention of some malignancies.

Berberine Nopal is found in the naturally occurring berberine. Several herbs, such as barberry (Berberi Vulgaris), have a long history of therapeutic usage and have a broad spectrum of antibiotic activity. In Ayurvedic and Chinese medicine.

Berberine has antibacterial, antiviral, antifungal, antiprotozoal, and antiworm action. It is frequently used to prevent many different forms of infections, particularly eye infections and bacterial diarrhea. Berberine and goldenseal extract have been shown in recent research to be highly inhibited by influenza.

Andrographis

Andrograph is a herbal stimulant that has been shown in multiple human clinical trials to lessen the severity of symptoms (particularly pain in the neck), as well as expectoration, nasal discharge, headache, fever, pain fish soup, malaise/fatigue, and sleep disturbances.

A multicenter research, which included John Hopkins, discovered that "herbal remedies are at least as effective as Rifaximin, with a "identical response rate and safety profiles." Dr. Logan had employed solvent mint oil (ECPO) on a patient with mild outcomes in a previous study. This is just one of many studies demonstrating the efficacy of the medications. You may see for yourself in the video below how antibiotics compare to herbal remedies and vitamins.

Were medications are also useful for managing the negative effects of antibiotics.

They could include the following items:

Sinus congestion is chronic Tiredness, heaviness, or fog Recurrent sinus or bladder infections Urgency or pressure to urinate Yeast infection that is chronic Stool that is loose, bloating, or a loss of appetite Nausea or vomiting Diarrhea or abdominal pain

Here are some additional measures to help you take care of your body when taking antibiotics: Probiotics-restore the body's healthy bacteria.

Anti-nausea herbal tea

The antioxidant effect of milk thistle on the liver. Consume onions and Czech to help the liver and keep yeast at bay.

With omega-3 fatty acids, vitamins C and E, and Oregon grape root. Make sure you eat a well-balanced diet. Of course, both antibiotics and natural therapies have advantages and disadvantages.

These facts should be considered before selecting what path to choose.

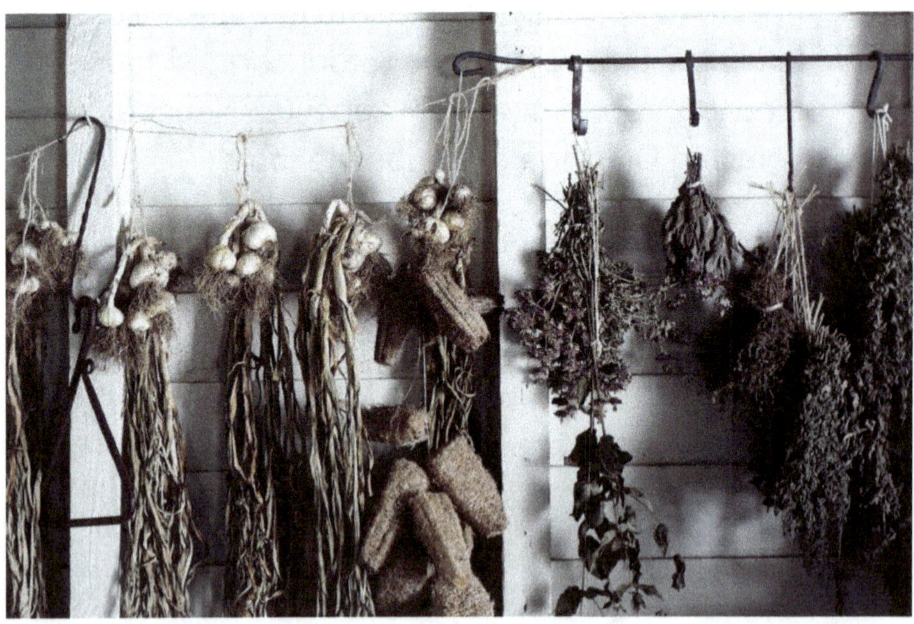

Antibiotic Advantages

The following are some of the most significant benefits of using antibiotics:

Antibiotics can treat a wide range of infections, including sore throat, tonsillitis, and sinusitis. Most antibiotics are simple to inject because I may administer them orally or intravenously.

There are numerous negative effects: many antibiotics have few side effects, making them an excellent choice when you are feeling extremely ill.

Cost effectiveness: most older forms of antibiotics, particularly those with generic counterparts, are generally quite affordable for any budget, even if you do not have health insurance.

Antibiotic disadvantages

Although antibiotics have many benefits, they also have a number of drawbacks, including:
Allergic reactions: Depending on your allergy medicine, you may be extremely allergic to certain antibiotics, such as those containing

sulfonamides. Unfortunately, because sulfur is contained in many common antibiotics, finding a good solution for your ailment may be more challenging.

Resistant bacteria: if you do not take the complete dose of antibiotics, you may only kill some of the bacteria in your system and become antibiotic resistant, which means that antibiotics may no longer work for you in the future.
While many antibiotics have a variety of side effects, some may induce unpleasant stomach problems, pain, nausea, diarrhea, and light sensitivity.

Furthermore, a Finnish study found that the effects of antibiotics on gut flora were detectable after a year. That is, the following antibiotic side effects are detrimental for a long period. Antibiotic misuse will result in the growth of resistant germs and more pointless death; therefore, if possible, we should utilize herbal antibiotic therapy.

Natural medicines have numerous advantages.

Unlike pharmaceutical preparations, there are a number of advantages to using herbal medicines:
Reduced risk of side effects: most herbal treatments are well-tolerated by patients and have fewer negative side effects than prescriptions. Herbs, on average, have fewer side effects than traditional medicine and may be safer to use over time.

Effective for chronic diseases: Herbal medications are more effective for long-term health issues that do not react well to standard medicine. Herbs and medications used to treat arthritis are examples of these. Vioxx, a well-known prescription medicine intended to treat arthritis, is remembered for increasing the risk of cardiovascular problems. Alternative arthritis remedies, on the other hand, entail a number of negative effects. Changes in diet, such as the addition of simple herbs, the elimination of nightshade vegetables, and the reduction of white sugar consumption, are examples of such treatments.

Lower cost: Another benefit of Phytotherapy is its low cost. Herbs are far less expensive than prescription medications. Prescription medicine costs are greatly increased by research, testing, and marketing. Herbs are typically less expensive than pharmaceuticals. Another advantage of herbal medicines is their widespread availability. Herbs can be obtained without a prescription. Simple herbs, such as mint and chamomile, can be grown at home. Herbs may be the sole therapy available to most people in some isolated places of the world.

Natural therapies have drawbacks

Herbs do have downsides, and Phytotherapy is not appropriate in all instances. The following are some disadvantages that must be considered:

Ineffective for a wide range of conditions: modern medicine addresses sudden and serious diseases and accidents far more effectively than herbal or other remedies. An herbalist would not be able to cure a severe trauma, such as a broken limb, or heal appendicitis or a heart attack as effectively as a conventional doctor employing current diagnostic testing, surgery, and medications. Another disadvantage of Phytotherapy is the very real danger of injury from self-dosing with herbs. Although it might be claimed that the same thing can happen with pharmaceuticals, such as an accidental overdose of cold medicine, many herbs do not come with instructions or packing information. Overdoes are a genuine possibility.

Poison risk connected with wild plants: gathering herbs in nature is dangerous, if not dangerous, however, some individuals attempt to identify and collect wild herbs. If they did not accurately identify the grass or used the wrong section of the plant, they would be poisoned.

Drug interactions: Herbal therapies can interact with prescription medications. Almost all herbs come with a warning, and many, such as anxiety-relieving herbs like valerian and St. John's wort, can interact with prescription medications like antidepressants. To avoid dangerous interactions, it is critical to discuss herbal medicines and supplements with your doctor.

Lack of regulation: Because plant products are not strictly regulated, buyers run the danger of purchasing inferior herbs. The quality of plant products can vary depending on the batch, brand, or manufacturer. This can make prescribing the correct dose of grass considerably more challenging.

These lists demonstrate why herbal antibiotics have been used for millennia – a long period, as compared to what modern antibiotics have developed. I have a job.

Because our bodies are combating bacteria and illnesses, we have considerably fewer adverse effects. Even when antibiotics are required by prescription, herbal remedies are excellent for keeping a healthy body and combating any side effects that may emerge.

BREAKING THE ANTIBIOTIC CYCLE

You have a sinus infection or a bladder infection; you seek medical attention and are prescribed an antibiotic; after discontinuing the prescription, do your symptoms return after seeing the doctor for additional antibiotics? Before you know it, your symptoms haven't gone away, and you've been taking many antibiotics for longer and longer lengths of time. Or do you take an antibiotic every day to try to keep infection symptoms at bay?

You're not alone, unfortunately. Antibiotics are the most commonly prescribed medications in the United States, with around 84 million written prescriptions written each year during office visits and 40 million prescriptions written after hospital discharge (CDC, The Hague). The Centers for Disease Control and Prevention estimates that just 10% of these antibiotic prescriptions are guaranteed.

The three most common sources of infection...

Not all infections are the same, despite the fact that they appear to give the same general symptoms: discomfort, swelling, redness, discharge, fever, soreness, and general weariness. The agents that induce infection, on the other hand, differ:

Virus. Viruses are little fragments of genetic code that enter a sensitive cell and take over its functions, causing the cell to produce more viruses. When viruses are recognized, the immune system promptly kills them. Viruses have "their period," which indicates that each virus has a regular delay in causing disease symptoms before the immune system eliminates it. Viruses cause almost 75% of all ear, sinus, and upper respiratory tract infections.

Mushroom. A mold is a form of fungi. Everyone's body contains a unique type of fungus (in the ears, nose, vagina, bladder, intestines, and intestines). Candida albicans is the culprit. This fungus must be present in order to protect the body and aid digestion in the intestines. When there is too much Candida, it might cause infection.

According to the Mayo Clinic, Candida infections account for 98 percent of all recurring infections and roughly 15 percent of new infections.

Bacterial. Bacteria are self-contained cells. They grow and create more bacterial cells when they enter a sensitive part of the body. A good immune system can kill bacteria; but, if the immune system is weak, a bacterial infection can persist. Bacterial infections account for around 10% of all infections.

Parasite. These are included because parasitic infections are possible. This type of infection is most commonly caused by raw pork products. Some scientists believe that everyone in the world has a parasitic infection and that parasites have caused many health problems. However, many patients show no indications of parasite infection. Parasites are responsible for less than 1% of infections.

Antibiotics and How They Work

Antibiotics are classified into 17 different groups, but they all act in the same way. Each antibiotic is either broad-spectrum ("broad spectrum") or specialized ("concentrated"). A broad-spectrum antibiotic is intended to kill a wide range of microorganisms. A focused antibiotic only kills one or two microorganisms. If you did not have a test before being prescribed an antibiotic, you would have received a broad-spectrum antibiotic;

practically all antibiotics supplied are broad-spectrum.

It is important to note that antibiotics have an effect on bacteria. Bacteria are self-contained cells. Our bodies are made up of many different types of cells. Cells are independent units in the body that are separated from one another by a shell. The shells of bacteria differ from the shells of our body's cells. As a result, the immune system is able to look for and recognize what is not a part of the body.

An antibiotic can accomplish the same thing. When a person takes an antibiotic, he seeks shells with a specific identity and eliminates these cells by cutting a hole in the bacteria's shell. As the cell dies, so do the bacteria.

Unfortunately, broad-spectrum antibiotics are incapable of distinguishing between healthy bacteria and those that cause infection. Our bodies include bacteria that are required for food digestion, vitamin and mineral absorption, and the nutritional mucosa. When an antibiotic is effective, it also kills these microorganisms.

(It should be noted that there are different "antibiotics" for parasitic illnesses (such as Actelion), viral infections (such as Tamiflu), and fungal infections) (such as Mycostatin or Lamisil). These are not the ones described in this article because they are rarely and infrequently prescribed.)

What about other sources of infection?

Antibiotics are exclusively effective against bacteria and will not work against viruses, fungi, or parasites. If you use an antibiotic for a virus, parasite, or fungal infection, the infection will not improve.

However, taking an antibiotic makes me feel better.

Illness symptoms are actually indicators that the immune system is combating the infection. Because a new, more hazardous substance has entered the body when an antibiotic is administered, the body's mending efforts are halted. Infection is bad (which is why your body was battling it), but hazardous substances are more destructive, therefore dealing with them takes precedence for your body's health. Even if the infection is caused by a virus, the symptoms of such an infection will diminish or disappear since the body's attention is diverted to something more dangerous. Remember that the symptoms of an illness are the immune system's response to infection. Without an immune system to combat infection, symptoms will diminish or disappear until the drug is eliminated or "managed" by the body.

Is it safe to take antibiotics on a regular (chronic) basis?

Aside from allergic reactions to antibiotics, there are numerous reported occurrences of adverse reactions, the most prevalent of which are diarrhea and nausea. Good bacteria in the digestive tract (intestines and stomach) aid in digestion and nutrient absorption. When the antibiotic kills these beneficial bacteria, digestion is disturbed, and the good yeast (Candida albicans) that lives in the intestine has more area to flourish. Remember that antibiotics do not destroy yeast. Not only is there an excess of yeast development, but there may also be a decrease in nutrient absorption and difficulties in breaking down the consumed food, resulting in diarrhea and the risk of nutritional deficiencies.

Immune suppression is a less-commonly discussed side effect. As previously said, when the body is confronted with chemical poisons or foreign substances, the immune system slows down. If a person is infected with a virus, the virus will continue to do more than itself, unaffected by an immune system. When the antibiotic is stopped, the virus resurfaces, but it is stronger because it has the opportunity to take a stronger bite. Furthermore, the fungal infection mentioned in the preceding paragraph will worsen throughout the antibiotic; it was also unaffected by an immune system. With yeast present throughout the body, it is probable that symptoms of recurring infection, such as sinusitis or bladder infection, are caused by yeast. As previously stated, the Mayo Clinic believes that 98 percent of recurrent infections are caused by yeast rather than bacteria, therefore repeating antibiotics would not have helped the condition.

Chronic infections have been linked to chronic fatigue syndrome as a result of scarring responses decreased by chronic antibiotic treatment.

Autoimmune illnesses are a new source of worry. It has been proposed and is currently being researched that consuming stimulating supplements while taking antibiotics increases the likelihood of getting an auto- immunological condition since the immune system becomes confused when inhibited and stimulated at the same time.

Another issue with long-term antibiotic use (which will not be explored here) is the emergence of "superbugs," bacteria that are resistant to antibiotics because they have been exposed to them so frequently that they have become "immune" to them.

What is the best way to break the cycle?

The immune system is meant to detect and eliminate any invader, whether bacterial, viral, parasitic, fungal, or otherwise. The more powerful the immune system, the quicker the response to these alien invaders.

What should I do?

Remember that diseases do not originate in a vacuum, thus there is no reason why a sickness affects and can persist. Always evaluate the emotions elicited by the condition, as well as the emotions that may have precipitated the difficulties. Each part of the body has different feelings; for example, the bladder is terrified, while the nose is sad and depressed.

Examine your living and working situations as well. Do you live in a moldy house if you have a recurrent sinus infection? Do you work in an area that has recently been repainted? Examine your personal habits. Do you frequently retain your bladder so that you only go to the toilet twice a day? Smoke?

It's also a good idea to add probiotics to your diet, such as acidophilus. Antibiotics, which eliminate beneficial microorganisms in the body, necessitate their replacement. There are several acidophilic or probiotic formulae on the market, or you can eat one yogurt per day with "live yogurt crops."

What do you think?

If you wish to break the antibiotic cycle and end your suffering, know that it is possible! You experience infection symptoms because your body is battling to get rid of it, which means all you have to do is help it along and the body will do the rest. You don't have to suffer for the rest of your life; you don't have to sacrifice your life, creativity, and joy because of a chronic infection. Recognize that you have choices. Recognize that you have the ability to be free of your sufferings.

Chapter 4: HERBAL REMEDIES TO PREVENT SERIOUS ILLNESS CAUSED BY ANTIBIOTICS

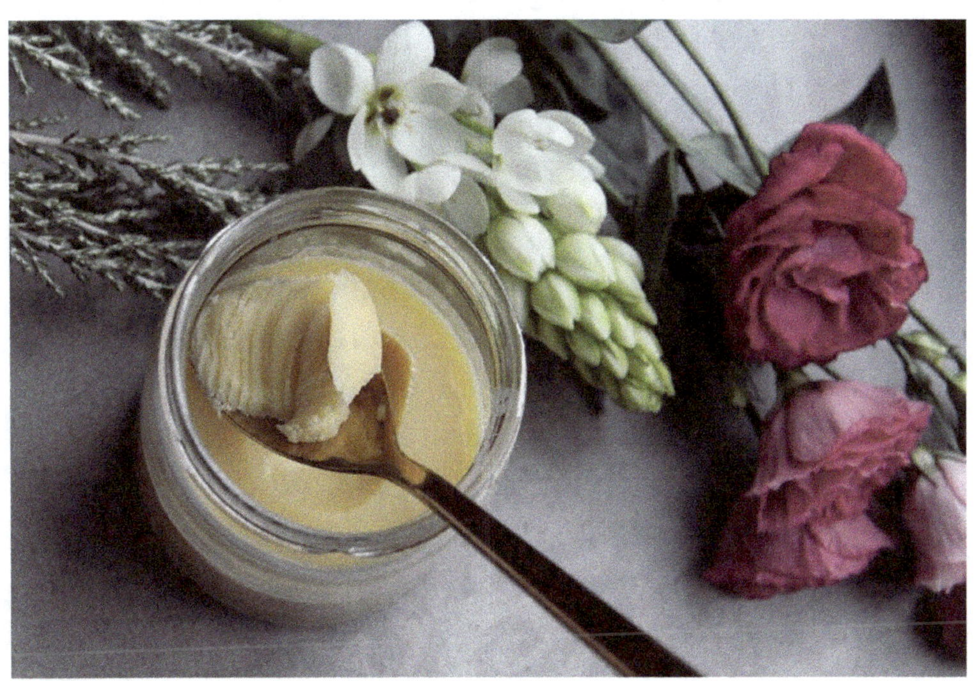

There are numerous definitions of insanity. One of them is a person's inability to comprehend the nature and repercussions of his actions. Another possibility is that the individual is a danger to himself or herself or others. Another is that the person clothes in a white gown and runs down the street screaming, "Help, the world is on fire."

People believe that if people take a herb, a plant, rather than a prescription pill, herbal therapy will be ineffective. Herbal treatments, according to many, were developed by God, while medications were produced by mortals. Who has the most clout? If you don't believe that herbs may be really potent, try a hemlock salad. Then take two aspirins and call me first thing in the morning.

Antibiotics were dubbed the "greatest stride forward since the advent of the mp3 player" when they were found. They were referred to as Caesar. Salad. Antibiotics killed microorganisms and kept many people alive who might otherwise have died. That is why, in the last two thousand years, the Earth's population has risen from one million to six billion. It is expected to reach 9 billion by 2050 when we will have consumed all of the herbs and will be forced to rely solely on artificial food. When Karl Benz invented the vehicle 150 years ago, it was considered the greatest invention since Lana Turner at the soda stand. We would not attack the Middle East for their oil if vehicles did not exist, and climate gases would not melt the Arctic and Antarctica. The sea level would not have risen by 50 feet, and Kevin Costner would not have blown up a parcel on Waterworld. Who would have guessed?

The bad news is that antibiotics have extremely harmful side effects. Consider your body to be a huge salad dish. Please take my salad bowl. Please. There are white flakes, your healthy bacteria, your flora and fauna, black weeds, bad bacteria, and harmful germs inside this salad dish. The antibiotic kills microorganisms in the stomach, intestines, and bloodstream. The bad news is that it also destroys beneficial microorganisms, such as white flakes. After a week of antibiotics, only black weeds, mushrooms, and yeast remain in your salad dish. These yeast fungi are living organisms that have their own population boom. They quickly take possession of your colon and proceed to eat their way through it into the bloodstream, which then absorbs every cell in your body. The Candida yeast then proceeds to coat and eat away at your organs, causing you to develop all of the diseases listed in the book. When there is no treatment, an ounce of prevention is worth a pound of cure.

You may experience melancholy, weariness, yeast infections, and emphysema, a condition in which your lungs resemble Swiss cheese and you sit in agony in a wheelchair with a mask hooked to the oxygen cylinders. Thank you very much, Dr. Frankenstein. You can't believe your doctor would do something like this to you. If not, inquire as to why doctors provide Paxil to suicidal patients when they are well aware that Paxil increases the patient's proclivity to commit suicide. Or you can inquire as to why your mailbox is flooded with Viagra advertisements while your doctor is well aware that Viagra causes blindness. The list of prescription medication side effects that cause short- and long-term death is enormous. It's all about the money. That is why Jesus destroyed the money changers' tables and referred to the Holy Temple as a den of thieves. Your neighborhood pharmacy is not a holy place. It is not even possible to find it in Jerusalem.

Antibiotics are sometimes quite effective in killing bacteria that are going to kill you. If you must take them, begin taking acidophilus after you have finished. Acidophilus tablets are packed with billions of beneficial bacteria. These beneficial bacteria can also be found in yogurt. These herbal cures, flora, and fauna begin to multiply, filling your salad bowl with nutritious white flakes while keeping the black weeds at bay. Take grapefruit seed extract pills to destroy black weeds as well. The most crucial thing is to use oregano.

Oregano is nature's most potent antibiotic. The oregano Herbal Remedy has been clinically proved to eliminate bacteria, viruses, mold, fungi, yeast, and black weeds in your salad bowl that even the strongest antibiotics cannot. Oregano is offered in a variety of forms as herbal medicine. It is available in natural food stores as oregano oil and oregano capsules. You can use the dropper to place it straight beneath your tongue or in a small amount of grapefruit juice. The advantage of oregano is that it does not kill white flakes. Instead, as it destroys Black weeds, it promotes their development.

Sinusitis affects a large number of people. Sinusitis is frequently caused by molds that are naturally present in the air we breathe, as well as bacteria, fungi, and parasites in the sinus cavities. Oregano frequently destroys them while also healing sinusitis. Allergies affect a large number of children and adults. Often, mold in the lungs is caused by airborne mold. Oregano, along with sage and cumin, other herbal medicines in the same pill, enters the bloodstream and kills the mold that reproduces in the lungs, destroying the source of Allergy and putting an end to asthma, bronchitis, and emphysema.

Millions of people are trapped in a never-ending cycle. A drug causes new ailments, which necessitate new drugs, which necessitate new drugs, and so on until you're standing at the pharmacy counter with a bag full of pills, in dreadful suffocating anguish, until death. Large pharmaceutical corporations do not advertise oregano since it grows in nature, they cannot patent it, and they cannot profit from it. This isn't to say you shouldn't go to your local health food store or order these herbal medicines right now to get rid of your toxic black weeds and start growing your flora and fauna.

Chapter 5: OUR IMMUNE SYSTEM

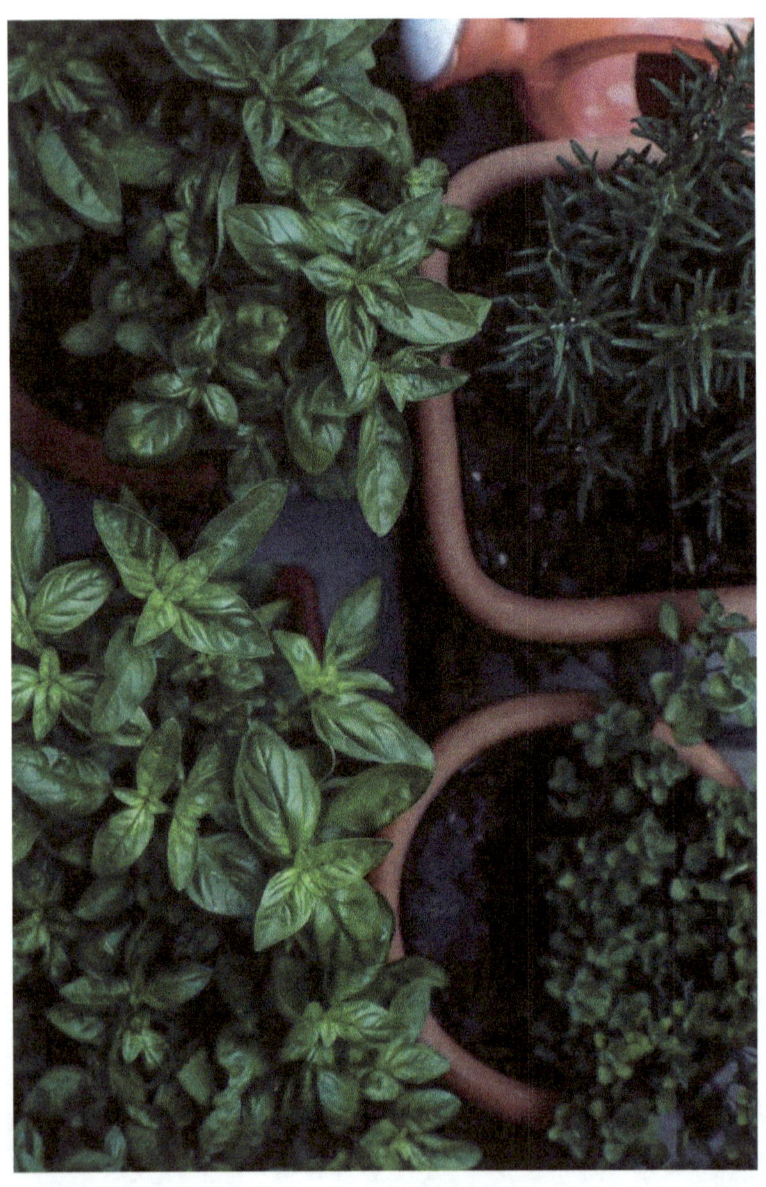

The immune system is a sophisticated humming mechanism. It preserves the basic ability to recall previous illnesses and prevents the body from succumbing to stress and illness. Furthermore, it features an improved communication system that gives the essential response to an infection or wound reaction. Immune cells provide the necessary secretions, which enhance the "fighting" immune cells. However, the immune system of the body may decrease, resulting in gout illness. It boosts immunity through eating healthily, resting well, exercising, spending time in the sun, and lowering stress.

As previously stated, synthetic antibiotics can effectively suppress the immune system, eradicating healthy bacteria and allowing the growth of hazardous bacteria in the presence of a weakened immune system. To keep your immune system in good shape, look for the immunostimulant herbs listed below. By strengthening the stomach, the immune system is enhanced. Malnourished persons are more likely to contract diseases over the world, as research has shown. As a result, it is critical to supplement your diet with the following herbs.

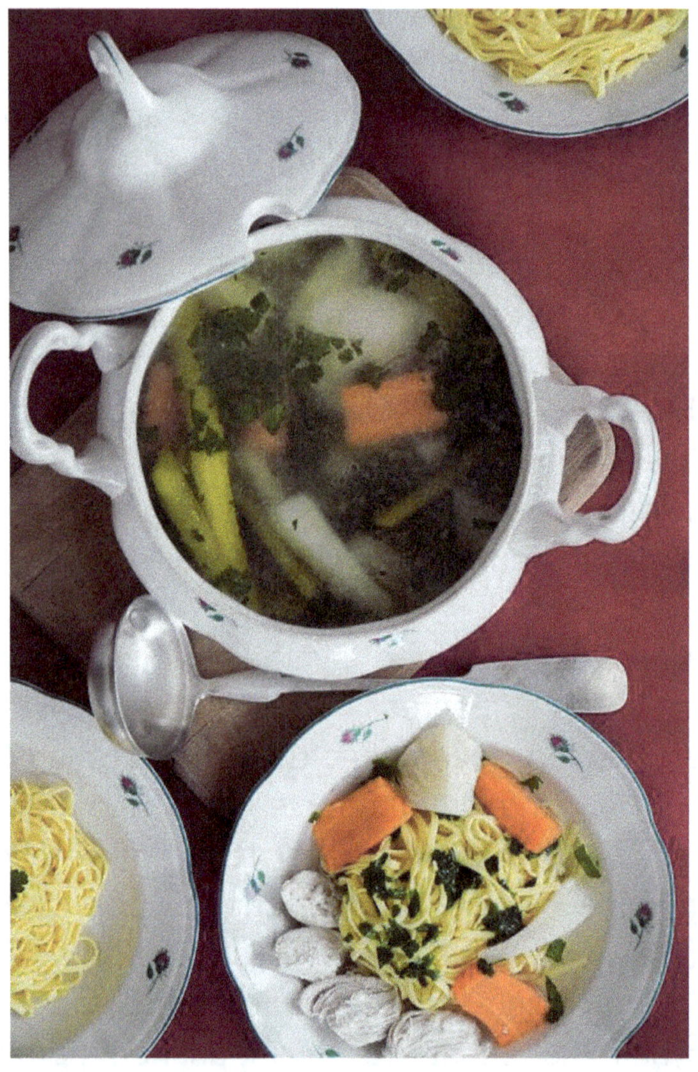

GINSENG

Ginseng can be found in a variety of forms all around the world. The most popular is Panax ginseng, also known as Korean ginseng. Ginsenoside, its primary component, has anti-inflammatory and anti-tumor properties. Protects the immune system and repairing cells from free radicals in the environment or poor dietary choices. Furthermore, it is recognized to fight diabetes.

Ginseng-Infused Asian Chicken Soup

Note: This recipe is great for repairing and treating the spleen and stomach, as well as strengthening the immune system. It makes use of root fibers, which are tiny strands that fall from the ginseng plant's main root.

Gross:

- Four chicken thighs
- Fivered dates, 10 g of ginseng fiber two slices of ginger root one tsp. salt
- Six cups of water

Instruction:

To begin, separate the chicken thighs into two pieces. Bring two cups of water to a boil in a saucepan, then cook the chicken for thirty seconds in the water. The chicken should then be removed from the boiling water and drained.

In a separate safe, heat-resistant bowl, combine the chicken, ginseng, dates, ginger root, and water. Spray the dish's components together in a steamer or a wok over boiling water. Continue to heat for two hours, resuming the water supply as soon as it evaporates. Remove the soup from the heat after two hours and serve hot.

Ginger

Ginger, a rough and unappealing root has anti-inflammatory effects. Ginger actually serves to prevent the inflammatory response of specific genes. Inflammation is the leading cause of all diseases in the body, including cancer, diabetes, and colds. Because cellular inflammation is minimized, it actively defends against future diseases. Furthermore, ginger aids in the prevention of blood clots, hypercholesterolemia, and cardiovascular disease.

Tartare of Tuna with Ginger Pepper Folder:

a pair of onions 1 pound tuna

1 ginger root, 1 inch red pepper flakes 6 tbsp soy sauce 1 tablespoon honey

2 tbsp sesame oil 1 lime juice 4 slices of bread

Begin with the tuna preparation. We cut the tuna into cubes and remove all of the bleeding line's dark sections. Place the tuna in a big bowl and keep it fresh.

Prepare the vegetables: red pepper, onion, and ginger root, all chopped. Mix in the onions, chili, and ginger with the tuna.

Mix together the soy sauce, lime juice, honey, and sesame oil on the side. Pour this mixture over the tuna and continue to whisk.

In a toaster or on a plate, toast each piece of bread. For a delectable experience, serve tartar on bread or directly on the side of toast.

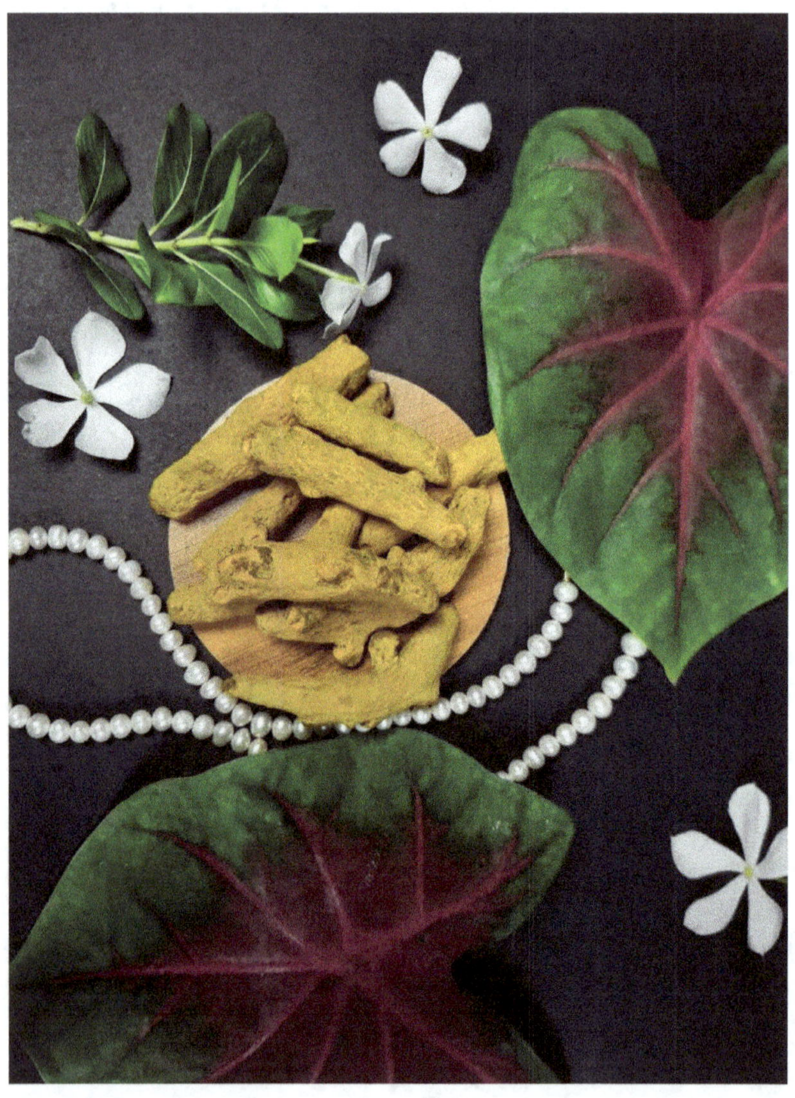

Turmeric

Turmeric is a curcumin-rich ancient Indian plant. Curcumin is high in antioxidants, which help to combat inflammation generated by free radicals in the body. Furthermore, it soothes the stomach by boosting bile flow and protects against bacterial infections. Turmeric stimulates the adrenal glands in the body, causing them to produce more hormones, which lowers symptoms of internal inflammation. Other studies demonstrate that turmeric protects the liver better, therefore it could be a toxin resulting from the high consumption of alcohol associated with turmeric use.

Tea with ginger and turmeric

The revitalizing effects of turmeric and ginger relieve internal discomfort and boost the immune system.

Folder:

14 teaspoon ground turmeric 14 teaspoon ginger 1 tablespoon soy milk

1 tsp. z. From. honey Instructions:

Begin by bringing water from the Cup to a boil in a bowl. Reduce the heat to low and add the turmeric and ginger. Allow the water and ingredients to come to a boil for around 10 minutes. So add the milk and thoroughly mix it in. Pour the mixture into a cup of tea and sweeten it with honey.

The Western Wonder Folder's Turmeric:

- 1 tablespoon oil
- 14 to 16 oz. tofu
- 12 cup crushed red pepper 14 cups sliced white onion 14 teaspoon coriander.
- Anaheim 12 Cup Pepper 14 teaspoon garlic powder 14 tsp cumin 1 12 tsp z. turmeric.
- 12 teaspoon z. From. Salt.

Direction:

To begin, remove the tofu from its package and place it on a dry cloth. Dry with paper towels until all of the water has been gone. Then, place it in a basin and crush it with a fork. Tofu should crumble.

Heat the olive oil in a medium-sized frying pan on the side. Prepare the chili, white onion, and Anaheim pepper by cutting and cutting into cubes after they have been heated for a bit. Put them in the oil. Cook, stirring periodically, for four minutes.

Then whisk in the cumin, coriander, garlic powder, and salt to the pepper-onion combination for one minute. Toss in the tofu and turmeric. Cook for another two minutes, then season with salt & pepper to taste. This meal can be eaten on its own or with warmed tortillas and avocado accompaniments.

Ganoderma

This Asian herb tastes like a bitter mushroom. It has been used in Chinese medicine for millennia, and new studies demonstrate that it boosts immunity and fights the early stages of cancer. It also contains antioxidants, which provide internal relaxation while reducing inflammation in the body. Consider this plant, especially if you want to relieve pain from urinary tract infections. Drinking tea with reishi mushrooms is the greatest method to reap the benefits of Ganoderma.

Tea with Reishi Mushrooms

Folder:

5 gram dried reishi mushrooms (try the brand Mountain Rose Herb from the local grocery store) three quarts water

Direction:

Breaking Ganoderma is extremely difficult; many claim that the procedure is similar to breaking coffee grinders or food processors. Make do with what you've got. Try a hefty blade or, more gingerly, your fingers. Alternatively, you can purchase a ready-made reishi bag.

Three cups of water should be brought to a boil. Reduce the temperature of the hob to a low setting after adding the mushroom pieces to the boiling water. Allow two hours for the water to boil. So strain the water and set the tea aside. Allow the tea to cool for a few minutes before sipping. Tea can be kept in the refrigerator for up to three days.

Claw of the Cat

Peruvian grass, sometimes known as a cat's claw, is commonly used to alleviate gastrointestinal disorders. Recent use, on the other hand, has been demonstrated to boost the immune system. It boosts the immune system, allowing for the secretion of a bigger number of fighting cells. Furthermore, the cat's claw contains oxindole alkaloids, which improve the body's ability to absorb and eliminate germs and viruses.

Immunity-Boosting Antiviral Tea

It's worth noting that this immunity-boosting tea also contains chuchuhuasi, which is proven to help patients with joint pain.

Gross:

- 1 teaspoon vanilla
- 1 tablespoon Goji Berries
- 12 teaspoon Bercampuri 1 tablespoon cat claw
- 12 tbsp chuchuhuasi Directions:

First, bring two liters of water to a boil in a pot, then immerse all of the ingredients in the boiling water. Allow the water to simmer for 10 minutes on low heat. The ingredients are then soaked and served hot.

Ginkgo Biloba (Ginkgo Biloba)

With the usage of the herb ginkgo biloba, you can say goodbye to vexing free radicals in the body caused by the external environment or bad nutrition. Gingko biloba leaves include bilobalides and ginkgolides, which act as antioxidants and anti-inflammatory agents. Furthermore, it was discovered that these qualities minimize radiation damage. According to recent research, the herb neutralizes free radicals, which cause cell death due to radiation; additionally, ginkgo lowers brain cell damage by roughly 50%.

Herbal Ginkgo Tea

Gross:

1 teaspoon dried ginkgo biloba 1 cup water

To begin, heat 1 cup of water. Pour in the dried herbs when it begins to boil. Boil water for twenty minutes on low heat. Then pour in the water and set aside to cool in a cup of coffee for a few minutes. Drink while it's still hot.

Rosemary

The exquisite perfume and evergreen nature of this Mediterranean shrub have long been loved by the ancient Greeks and Romans. Plant rosemary boosts the immune system and promotes blood circulation, allowing oxygen to enter the body's cells more quickly. The brain is powerful, with a strong focus. Furthermore, the increased blood flow helps digestion and lessens the severity of an asthma episode.

- Rosemary Roasted Sweet Potatoes with Razzmatazz:
- Six massive sweet potatoes

- 12 cup sprigs fresh rosemary 12 cups extra-virgin olive oil 1 teaspoon pepper
- 1 tablespoon salt

Instruction:

To begin, preheat the oven to 325 degrees Fahrenheit. Cut the potatoes into fried components by cutting them lengthwise. Place the fried quarters on a baking sheet and drizzle with the remaining 1/3 cup olive oil. Then season the chips with rosemary, salt, and pepper to taste.

Place the baking tray in the oven and bake for 10 minutes, turning the chips halfway through. Cook the chips for another 20 minutes.

Water the sweet potatoes with the remaining olive oil before serving.

YEAST INFECTION NATURAL REMEDIES

Candida albicans, often known as candidiasis, is one of the most perplexing to medical research, affecting millions of women and men worldwide who suffer from this state of unconsciousness on a regular basis. Debilitating symptoms of yeast infections are produced by fungal proliferation, which occurs in a variety of diseases and varies in severity. Although some doctors have prescribed antibiotics for this ailment, research investigations have shown that herbs for yeast infections outperform pharmaceutical treatment in the majority of cases.

One issue is that Candida albicans is not foreign to the human body; it is a yeast fungus that regularly coexists with other bacteria. When the development rate of this fungus becomes uncontrollable, it causes thrush; infections that appear as white spots on the tongue, in the mouth, and in the throat, making chewing and swallowing uncomfortable.

One of the most prevalent causes of Thrush in adults is the use of antibiotics, which, unfortunately, kill not only dangerous bacteria but also lactobacilli, which the body requires to keep the fungus Candida albicans under control. The fungus grows in the presence of high quantities of glucose in the saliva; people who smoke, wear dentures or have diabetes are more likely to get oral thrush.

Women who use oral contraceptives are more likely to develop vaginal yeast infections, and thrush can occur during pregnancy. It is easily transmitted from mother to child during childbirth or breastfeeding due to its adaptability. Yeast infection, with its vast range of symptoms, might go undiagnosed in parts of the body such as joints and intestines.

Candida albicans is also linked to a poor diet; the typical American diet, which is high in refined sugars and acidic foods, disrupts the pH balance in the intestine. Long-term stress increases the fungus's growth. Natural yeast infection treatments work best when combined with a good diet.

Herbs Used to Treat Candida Albicans Oregano (Origanum compactum):

Essential oil has a stimulating and warming effect and can be used internally or externally as a natural cure for yeast infections. Carvacrol and thymol, which are found in oregano oil, are responsible for its antibacterial and antifungal properties. Carvacrol has been demonstrated in studies to reduce the growth of Candida albicans. Oregano contains flavonoids, ursolic and oleanolic acids, vitamin A and vitamin C, and has antibacterial characteristics that have been shown to be effective against E. coli and Staphylococcus.

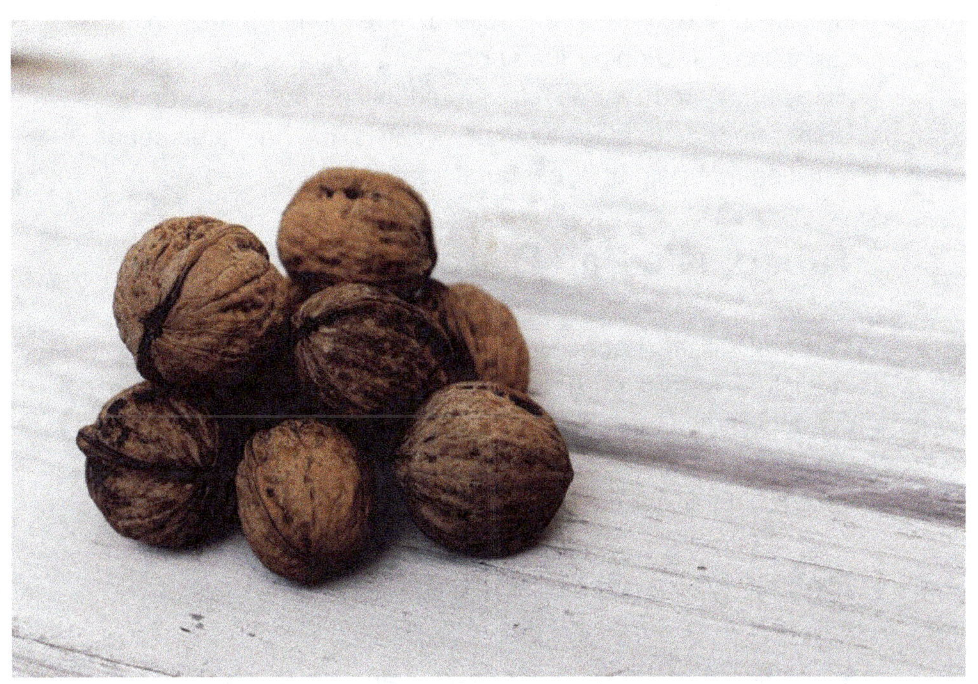

Juglans Nigra (Black Walnut):

Black walnut, one of the most potent herbs for yeast infections, is used as an antifungal agent as well as an antiseptic to treat and cure Candida albicans. Oxygenates the blood and is utilized to manage sugar levels as well as eliminate toxins and fats. Thrush (oral yeast infection), vaginitis (vaginal yeast infection), jock itch (yeast infection), and parasitic diseases are all treated with black walnut.
As a yeast herbal infection, black walnut is used to treat intestinal diseases caused by Candida albicans, including as irritable bowel syndrome (IBS), parasite infections of the intestine, and intestinal bacterial infections. It has high quantities of tannin, juglandin, and juglansacid and is utilized for both indoor and outdoor purposes. Organic iodine, found in black walnut green skin, has antiseptic qualities that help fight bacterial infections.

Tabebuia's Pau D'arco:

The bark of the Lapacho tree is used to make this Phyto-medicinal herbal cure for yeast infections. Pau D'arco's major active ingredient is lapachol, which inhibits mold growth and functions as a respiratory toxin for microbes, inhibiting their generation of oxygen and energy.

Neem (Azadirachta Indica) Leaves:

Because of its potent antibacterial and antifungal qualities, the neem tree is employed in Ayurvedic medicine. It is a bitter herb that contains the alkaloids Azadirachtin and

Nimbin. This herb for yeast infections is a wonderful cleanser for the skin and blood, and it is extremely effective in normalizing intestinal bacteria. Pregnant women should avoid using this herb.

Thor Sturluson is a Copenhagen-based amateur biologist and herbalist.

THE MOST EFFECTIVE HOME REMEDIES FOR URINARY TRACT INFECTION

What are the best home remedies for a urinary tract infection? Natural therapy works by helping the body to recognize and kill E. coli in the urinary system. But, before we get into these three cures, you should be aware that you must cease using medicines to treat the illness!

The Real Deal about UTI Antibiotics

Antibiotics are being abused! Listen to top experts and scientists discuss the use of antibiotics in the United States.

Dr. McDougal, a doctor, and nutritionist stated: "In today's environment, over-prescription and excessive use of psychotropic medicines cause far more harm than good. Often, only a few basic lifestyle changes are required, rather than pricey medicines with potentially deadly side effects. Unfortunately, most doctors do not advise us on easy lifestyle modifications, but I do not hesitate to prescribe one or two medications.

Done! If you are taking antibiotics to treat a urinary tract infection, you have a 25% chance of getting another infection over the next several months. Why?

Antibiotics treat urinary tract infections by either eliminating all of the bad and healthy bacteria in the urinary system or allowing bacteria to bind to each other in the urinary tract. Unfortunately, most ulcers and E. coli are becoming drug-resistant.

As a result, lots of individuals are turning to home cures for urinary tract infections. Here are some of the most commonly utilized remains in the treatment of E. coli.

Three natural cures for urinary tract infections

1. Many individuals use unsweetened cranberry juice as a quick treatment. Cranberry juice and pills have been gradually used in numerous procedures because the chemical in the fruit actually kills the germs and E. coli that are already clinging to the urinary system walls. During an attack, many sick people consume at least four glasses of juice every day.

1. Another good approach is to boost the immune system as soon as feasible. It is possible to restore vitamin C and zinc pretty well. These two will dramatically boost your immune system, allowing it to begin battling germs and coli. We recommend 3000 mg of vitamin C every day and at least three zinc tablets. Vitamin C tablets of 1000 mg should be taken three times each day.

1. The majority of people who effectively treat and prevent future episodes utilize a multi-ingredient solution that includes a herbal supplement. Alfalfa is a powerful herbal

medicine that should be tried. Alfalfa juice concentrates can increase kidney function, and it turns out that good kidney functions are vital for eliminating urinary tract infections. Alfalfa aids in the removal of toxins from the body and increases the flow of urine (and, hopefully, bacteria).

A natural UTI treatment that works in 12 hours!

It identifies and searches for a step-by-step home remedy for UTI that works in 12 hours or less, so kindly check our website immediately. Our medicine is doctor-approved and costs the same as food!

NATURAL ALTERNATIVES TO SEASONAL SICKNESSES - HERBAL ANTIBIOTICS

If you have a cold that you can't seem to shake, you might be shocked to realize that there are effective natural remedies accessible at any health food store or drugstore—knowing that you can save money on visits to the doctor and trips to the pharmacy.

Antibiotics from Herbs:

Natural plant antibiotics such as olive oil/extract are beneficial. Follow the directions on the vial and take it multiple times a day.

Another antibacterial that works well with it is colloidal silver. Always purchase colloidal money from a reliable provider and never exceed the suggested dose. If done correctly, this can be a very effective tool in the fight against many common ailments.

Grapefruit oil/extract is an antibiotic as well, however, it appears to be a little thicker than the olive leaf. It is preferable to hide from dangerous insects such as Streptococcus. But be warned: you must dilute it with fluids, and it tastes horrible. Pinch your nose, drink it quickly, and bring orange juice or something with a strong taste to drive it away. * Do not mistake with grape seed oil.

Oregano oil/extract is a good antibacterial as well, however, it is a little softer than the olive leaf. When the author's children are cold, he frequently takes them for a ride.

The duration of the antibiotic course is as follows:

Once you start taking antibiotics, I'm sure you're taking them for 10-14 days, even if you feel better sooner, simply to make sure the bug doesn't come back. If you've finished the course of antibiotics but are still not feeling well, don't start again straight away; instead, see another doctor or look for another treatment option.

"Bacon-Friendly Bacteria"

Monitor all antibiotics; of course, whether they are plant-based or not, we recommend replenishing "friendly" bacteria in your diet with items like yogurt (with live cultures), sauerkraut, or kimchi. Furthermore, you can achieve this simply by taking "probiotics," which are available in pill form in various health food stores (look in the fridge). Leaving the "good bacteria" after antibiotic treatment can result in a seemingly unrelated, but nevertheless severe yeast infection or fungal illness a few weeks later. Yes, people with fungi or "yeast infections" are also known as "athlete's foot" or "athlete's itch," to name a few examples, but there are many more types of diseases that can arise if your "good bacteria" and "bad bacteria" are out of balance. In any event, once you're out of the antibiotic cycle, count on getting a little per-biotika. Take cabbage for dinner several times a week, or even a small amount of yogurt for breakfast. BTW, Pro-biotics mode, as discovered, to successfully treat "bird flu," which should never explode and become a problem.

Final Thoughts:

Of course, the ideal option is Preventive Medicine - take care of yourself first and foremost, and avoid being sick. There is no pharmaceutical that can substitute a healthy diet, rest, exercise, and preventive measures. Take your vitamins, get plenty of exercises, and so forth. Antioxidants, for example, are a good method to enhance the immune system, if only marginally, but that's a different topic.

If you enjoyed this post and would want to engage in further debates regarding natural and alternative medicine, among other things, you are invited to visit the mountain forum, where we delve into many elements of the "mountain man" way of life.

Caution: like with any ongoing treatment, continue with caution. You can trust if (e) are adequately educated before taking pharmaceuticals or supplements, or see an Accredited Specialist. Before beginning treatment, ensure that the condition has been accurately diagnosed. Certain plants and chemicals cause allergies or intolerances in some people, therefore these plants or chemicals are not suitable remedies for people.

This post is intended to inform your readers about the possibilities of alternatives to common allopathic remedies. The author is not a medical practitioner and should not be misunderstood. Take the information provided here, investigate it for yourself, and use your best judgment in deciding how to apply it.

ANTIFUNGAL HERBAL REMEDIES

Antifungal medications and therapies are used to eliminate fungus and yeast that cause infections in a variety of organs.

These medications are used to treat common ailments such as athlete's foot, ringworm, dandruff, and vaginitis, as well as complex conditions that have spread throughout the body. Antifungal treatments are frequently used in persons who have a weakened immune system, as observed in people with AIDS and those using immune suppressing medications.

Fungal Infections Come in a Variety of Forms

The following are some of the most frequent types of fungal infections that affect and irritate many people.

- Athlete's foot is a fungal illness that most commonly develops between the toes but can also affect the toenails and the bottom or sides of the feet.

- Worm. A fungal infection of the hair, skin, or nails. Tinea usually starts as a little red patch the size of a pea on the skin. It expands in a circle or circle as it increases. This condition is usually referred to as ringworm because it resembles microscopic worms under the skin.
- Jock itch is a fungal illness that affects both men and women in the groin and upper thighs.
- Honest. This yeast infection resembles a fungus. It usually affects the skin surrounding the nails or soft and wet areas near the body's openings. Diaper rash in children can be caused by a candidiasis infection. Yeast infections are a type of candidal infection that can occur in and around the vagina in older girls and adults.

Antifungal Treatment using Herbs

- Garlic. This herb is thought to have potent antibacterial properties. Albert Schweitzer used it to treat amoebic dysentery, and Louis Pasteur employed it as an antibacterial agent. Garlic is one of the greatest sources of the element germanium, which is a strong inducer of interferon and can help fight cancer by modifying the immune response.

- Tea tree oil is an extract from the original tree that grows in Australia. This is a treatment for a variety of fungal diseases of the mucous membranes. Internally, it is used to treat thrush and esophagitis, while topically, it is used to treat fungal infections of the skin and nail bed. Tea tree oil and grapefruit seed extract can be used to treat candida-related skin illness externally by combining 2-3 drops of each in a lotion or balm and applying it to the affected area.

- Oregano. This herb extract is said to be more effective and less dangerous than Nystatin at eradicating the fungus. It is also thought to be more effective and less harmful in eradicating staphylococcal infections.

- Echinacea is an antibacterial and immunostimulant plant. According to scientific evidence, herbal antibiotics have cortisol-like activity and aid in wound healing, the creation of systemic interferon, and the stimulation of T cells.
- Pau d'arco This plant is derived from the bark of a South American tree and is well-known for its potent antifungal qualities.
- The prestigious Golden Seal. Because of its tonic effects on the mucous membranes, this plant is said to be effective in treating most digestive issues ranging from peptic ulcers to colitis. It is a strong antibacterial agent that improves all mucous membranes, particularly mucous membranes.

REMEDIES FOR HERBAL HEMORRHOID

Hemorrhoids are a prevalent issue that affects millions of people around the world. This is an ancient problem, and there is no reason to be embarrassed about it. There are numerous hemorrhoid treatments available, including surgery, allopathic therapies, homeopathy, and herbal cures. Thousands of people have been cured in all of these ways.

Herbal hemorrhoid medications, on the other hand, have grown in favor in recent years. People prefer natural therapies over surgery or antibiotics. The main reason for this shift is that these medications alleviate the discomfort, irritation, and inflammation produced by hemorrhoids. Popular herbs such as witch hazel, butcher's broom, aloe vera, and others offer great outcomes for sufferers while producing no other health issues.

Furthermore, herbs used as hemorrhoid cures aid in the treatment of various disorders that a person may be suffering from. Natural herbal substances are generally safe and well-tolerated by the human body. These herbs are affordable and easily obtained from a herb store. The sole disadvantage of herbs is that they do not have to produce quick results.

Some herbs are applied topically, while others can be taken orally as hemorrhoid medications. Some herbs can be applied locally as well as ingested orally. Aloe vera, for example, can be applied to swollen veins and taken orally. Treatment with herbal hemorrhoids usually yields excellent and long-lasting effects.

Another advantage of herbal hemorrhoids therapy is that it does not have to be in the form of pills or ointments. Herbs can also be included in your diet by including them in your cookery. Many herbs, including mint, coriander, ginger, and cumin seeds, are used in cuisine. Some of these herbs will help you get rid of constipation and enhance your bowel motions.

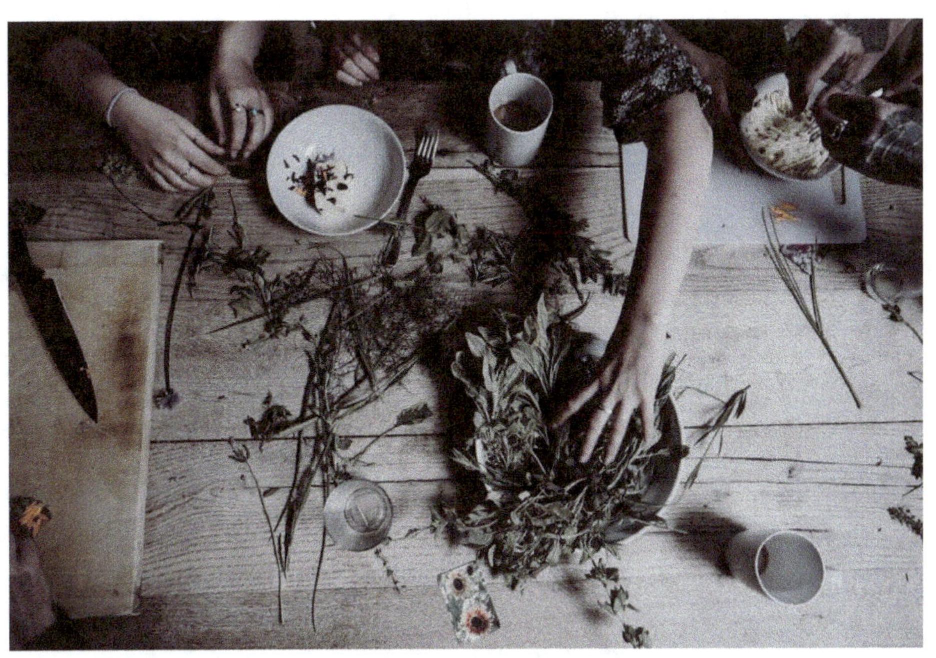

THE BV HERBAL REMEDY

After a positive diagnosis, BV (or bacterial vaginosis) should be treated as soon as possible. The removal of BV, whether via the use of antibiotics or a herbal cure, will avoid other issues that can affect fertility and pregnancy. Herbal therapies for BV are now widely recognized as the most effective and least intrusive type of treatment.

According to the World Organization for Women's Health, herbal remedies are now the most often used treatment for BV globally. In addition, in the United States in 2008, just under 35% of women with bacterial vaginosis used a herbal cure to treat their infection.

BV Facts and Herbal Remedies

BV is not an illness or something new that enters the body. It is caused by an increase in anaerobes, a type of bacteria already present in the vagina, and a decrease in lactobacilli, another type of bacteria.

This equilibrium results in a yellow/white film adhering to the vaginal walls and being released on a regular basis, with a nauseating odor, especially after sexual intercourse. In addition to discharge and odor, patients report severe vaginal irritation.

If the illness is left untreated for an extended period of time, physical complications may arise. Often, the most serious issues are psychological in nature. Women frequently experience embarrassment and create an adventure for sexual intercourse.

BV herbal therapies have a rate of clarity that approaches 100%, compared to 63 percent when antibiotics are used. They also tend to permanently cure the illness, whereas antibiotics have a high incidence of return.

Another significant advantage of using a herbal cure for BV is that there are no negative effects. Most of us are now aware of how much antibiotic use can harm the immune system. Herbal medicines, on the other hand, effectively aid develop the immune system while also removing vaginitis.

The ingredients for a herbal treatment for BV should not cost more than $4 or $5. You'll need a decent reference book that outlines the components and preparation, as well as the amount and frequency of use.
Drinking more water, not watering, staying dry and clean, avoiding scented personal hygiene products, and avoiding slightly looser cotton jeans and underwear are all healthy practices.

Once BV (bacterial vaginosis) has been diagnosed by the patient, a doctor, or a clinical counselor, it requires therapy. Natural BV solutions are the safest and most effective ways to get rid of BV.

According to the Institute for Women's Health and Wellness in Washington, DC, about 8% more women select BV natural therapies each year. The medical profession supports and encourages the use of BV herbal therapies, and antibiotics as treatment will become obsolete in the near future.

Bacterial vaginosis must be present in some form or another because it is capable of producing difficulties in addition to extreme itching and foul odor. Infections of the fallopian tubes and/or uterus can arise if left untreated. Pelvic inflammatory illness is frequent in BV patients who are untreated. PID can result in ectopic pregnancy and infertility. If bacterial vaginosis is present during pregnancy, abortions may occur.

Of course, it goes without saying that BV can keep a lot of women from having sex. It is usually at its worst after sexual contact, thus victims frequently abstain from sex to prevent extreme itching and disgusting fish odors.

Why should you avoid antibiotics in the treatment of bacterial vaginosis?

Antibiotics can be used there and were, until recently, the de facto treatment for BV. However, metronidazole and clindamycin have an effect on beneficial bacteria, which are necessary for a healthy immune system. Treatment can be lengthy, and a woman's health frequently deteriorates over time.

BV natural therapies, on the other hand, have no side effects and do not disrupt the body's natural balance. The incidence of clarification is also significantly higher with BV natural therapies, especially when combined with a certain diet. Treatment time is also greatly reduced. Furthermore, the immune system as a whole is strengthened. Many women prefer to stay on a natural path since they get sick less frequently and feel better overall.

Most BV treatments are inexpensive for a month's supply. You simply know what ingredients to use, how and in what quantities to combine them, and how and when to consume them. The primary recommendation is to obtain a proven guide BV natural remedies, so you know how to produce the remedy, what foods to avoid, and what diet to follow. In addition, you should think about frequent exercise and techniques to alleviate stress.